WITHDRAWN

Worldwatch Paper 9

The Two Faces of Malnutrition

Erik Eckholm
Frank Record

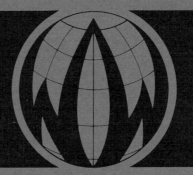

December 1976

Worldwatch Institute

Worldwatch Institute is an independent, non-profit research organization, created to identify and to focus attention on global problems. Directed by Lester R. Brown, Worldwatch is funded by private foundations and United Nations and governmental agencies. Worldwatch papers are written for a worldwide audience of decision makers, scholars, and the general public.

The Two Faces
of Malnutrition

Erik Eckholm
Frank Record

Worldwatch Paper 9
December 1976
3/22/85

The authors and Worldwatch Institute are grateful to the
United Nations Environment Program for supporting the
research for this paper, which is drawn from a forthcoming
book on environmental influences on health. This paper
may be partially reproduced with acknowledgement to
Worldwatch Institute. The views expressed are the responsibility of the authors and do not necessarily represent the
views of the manuscript reviewers; of Worldwatch Institute
and its directors, officers, or staff; or of the United Nations
Environment Program.

Printed on recycled paper

Table of Contents

Until quite recently, getting together enough food to stay alive was humanity's overriding dietary challenge. Today, hundreds of millions of people still need to worry about the same primal task. It isn't surprising, then, that the word "malnutrition" evokes images of pleading eyes and wasted bodies.

5

Underconsumption—what most people think of when they think of malnutrition—does promote disease and premature death. But malnutrition can result from an improper diet of any sort. In the present century, overconsumption has joined underconsumption as a medical scourge. Malnutrition today has more than one face.

Undernutrition and overnutrition have similar consequences for the individual: reduced life expectancy, increased susceptibility to disease, and reduced productivity. And the number of people afflicted by the modern plague of overnutrition is approaching that suffering undernutrition. In nearly every country in the world, rich or poor, malnutrition of one kind or another contributes to more deaths than does any other factor save, in some countries, age itself.

Both under- and overnutrition occur in visible extremes that, iceberg-like, only hint at the true magnitude of the human costs they entail. Gross underconsumption of the sort that shrivels bodies and often brings on rapid death is the sorry lot of tens of millions of children in poor countries. But many times more children, and numerous adults as well, live with less evident food deficiencies that subvert their health by abetting disease and that may impair their ability to learn and think. More than a quarter of all the world's deaths occur among children under five, and undernutrition has a hand in most of them.

For some of the world's better-off, a gross imbalance between food intake and physical activity fosters obesity, which in turn can lead

The authors wish to thank Professor Aaron M. Altschul, Professor Nevin S. Scrimshaw, Dr. Robert Morris, George Record, and Dr. Alan Waltman for reviewing the entire manuscript; Alan Berg, Dr. Joaquin Cravioto, and Dr. Jon E. Rohde for reviewing the sections on undernutrition; Dr. Junichi Iwai for reviewing the section on hypertension; and Dr. John W. Berg, Dr. Denis P. Burkitt, Dr. William Haenszel, and Dr. M. J. Hill for reviewing the section on diet and cancer.

to fatal heart disease, diabetes, and other disorders. But far more deaths, apparently including those caused by many cancers as well as by diseases of the circulatory system, are associated with the historically unprecedented intake of fats and refined foods by modern Western people—a dietary trend with consequences less visible than obesity. In the context of a sedentary lifestyle, the diet generally associated with prosperity—a diet rich in beef and other fatty livestock products —appears less the boon than the bane of affluence.

Doctors and drugs alone can seldom cure the diseases of malnutrition. Preventive measures are the sole effective means of control. In the poor countries this simple truth is well-understood. Over the last half decade, the concept of national nutrition planning has spread like good news through Africa, Asia, and Latin America. The speed and success with which such plans are being carried out certainly varies widely, but the idea of a national nutrition policy is now firmly entrenched in many poor countries.

In terms of nutrition strategies, the rich countries can learn something from the less developed world. In the West, economic development and, in some cases, government policies have gone a long way toward solving the historic problems of undernutrition. But almost all the industrial countries are woefully unprepared to combat the new forms of malnutrition associated with abundance. Outside of Scandinavia, the concept of a health-centered national nutrition policy has not yet caught on in the capitals of the developed countries.

Through educational, welfare, and agricultural programs, Western governments have long been deeply enmeshed in nutritional concerns, but in a haphazard, often inconsistent way. Thus in the United States, the Department of Agriculture actively promotes increased consumption of high-fat meats and cholesterol-heavy eggs, even as health officials in other federal agencies urge people to cut fat and cholesterol intake. The choice, then, is between this sort of wasteful contradiction and a coherent national nutrition policy that gives priority to public health over special interests.

One-twelfth of the U.S. national product is now devoured by the medical-care system. American health expenditures *grew* by more than a billion dollars a month in 1975, adding up to an annual total

of $115 billion. Health authorities assert almost unanimously that
money spent to eradicate the roots of disease will pay much greater
social returns than will extra billions poured into a costly curative
apparatus. And, with diet apparently a factor in more than half of all
deaths in the Western countries, the new stronghold of preventive
medicine must be the pantry.

7

The Human Geography of Undernutrition

The "world food crisis" has recently become headline-caliber news.
Aspects of this "crisis," however, have quietly haunted the back
pages for decades. The world food problem actually comprises numerous components, some old as civilization, some new as the 1970s, all
intermeshed, but each analytically distinct.

One aspect of the food problem that always rivets public attention is
famine. Modern communications, trade, and aid all help check the
local starvation that regional crop failures once heralded. But even
today when the harvest fails in destitute or isolated areas, or when
war disrupts food production and trade, famine may clench its bony
fist.

No image more effectively conjures a Malthusian nightmare among
the well-fed majority than does that of the gaunt faces of the starving.
Yet famine, however horrid and however photogenic, is in every case
a localized disaster whose impact can be warded off, sometimes entirely, by effective national and international planning. However, the
measures essential to forestall famines—early detection and aid—will
not combat other crucial components of the food problem.

Spectacular disruptions in the world's commercial food market since
1972 have probably generated even more public anxiety worldwide
than has famine. As the global demand for food surged past available
supplies, reserves were drawn dangerously low, prices multiplied as
they never had before, and food-surplus countries imposed unprecedented controls on food exports. Events demonstrated graphically
that the comfortable surpluses and stability of the postwar global
food market can no longer be taken for granted.

The horror of recent famines and the jolt of tripling grain prices have diverted attention from the most basic and widespread food problem of all: the chronic undernutrition suffered by the world's poor. Undernutrition is an invisible crisis, a daily tragedy that deprives hundreds of millions of the right to realize their genetic potential—their birthright. Pervasive and lasting, undernutrition does not make dramatic news copy, but its toll in human life far outweighs that of occasional famines.

The various aspects of the world's food problem are, of course, closely interconnected. Developments in one profoundly affect those in another. When grain reserves run low, for example, the international capacity to stave off imminent famines with food aid shrinks commensurately. When grain prices soar, the number of undernourished people soars as well. Those spending 60-80 percent of their income on food, as hundreds of millions do, can hardly offset a doubling in the price of grain by spending more. They must tighten their belts, even if they have no notches left.

But though undernutrition is intertwined with the commercial food market's crisis of supply, demand, and management, the two are not identical. Widespread undernutrition predated the food-market turbulence of the 1970s and, should government policies stabilize the food market, will outlast the storm. Even if our reserve bins overflow again, undernutrition will still have a firm hold. Undernutrition is a manifestation of poverty, one ultimately rooted in the political and economic structures that engender economic deprivation. These roots run deep indeed; they will not be totally eradicated by wise planning alone, but only through fundamental reforms of social institutions.

In any specific case, dietary deficiencies may be tied to various "causes." As victims of ignorance and superstition, people often fail to take full advantage of indigenous foods. Or, lured by advertisers and the examples set by wealthier women, mothers may switch their nursing infants from breast to bottle even though adequate quantities of commercial formulas are beyond their financial reach. Overcrowding as a result of a swelling population, inequitable land distribution, or both, leaves some rural families without enough land to feed themselves. Others are left with no land at all.

The list of factors linked to undernutrition fills many pages, but each factor is in some sense a manifestation of poverty. The poor, wherever they live, are susceptible to undernutrition; the rich, wherever they live, can purchase an adequate diet. The persistence of widespread undernutrition in a world that produces ample food for all can only be construed as a measure of the global social order's failure to satisfy basic human needs.

Perceptions of the scale and severity of undernutrition in the world have changed along with our data-gathering methods and our understanding of human dietary needs. The United Nations estimates of the protein requirements of a healthy person, for example, were scaled downward by about a third in the early 1970s, redefining and thereby eliminating much of the international "protein gap" perceived in earlier decades. Recent studies, however, suggest that the redefined protein standards may be too low; a group of U.S. university students fed the new "safe" level of protein developed signs of protein deficiency after two months.[1]

A related shift in scientific thinking stems from the emerging understanding of how protein and food energy interact in the body. Both are essential for body growth and maintenance, but when the body is short of calories, available protein is poorly utilized and may be burned as energy to make up the deficit. Thus, even though a patient may show overt signs of a protein shortage, the underlying problem may be more complex—a deficiency of energy, or protein, or both. In view of the possible protein-energy interactions, the general term "protein-calorie malnutrition" is now commonly used to describe the undernutrition of the poor.

From 1950 to 1970, official estimates of the extent of undernutrition in the world fell steadily. No one can say how much of the drop reflected true improvement in the nutritional state of humanity, and how much reflected changing definitions and improved statistical methods. All three factors probably came into play.

Several global surveys by the U.N. Food and Agriculture Organization and the U.S. Department of Agriculture in the first three decades after World War II reached the same conclusion: close to half of humanity suffered from a shortage of protein or calories or both. All these estimates, however, were based on questionable assumptions about consumption needs, and most of them relied on national food-consumption averages that ignored sub-national variations in food habits and income. In preparation for the 1974 World Food Conference, the United Nations reassessed the world nutrition situation using the latest notions of nutritional requirements, and, for the first time, considering rich as well as poor countries. This study found about 460 million people—or one in every six people included in the survey—to be undernourished as of 1970.[2]

Unfortunately, the U.N. study could not include data on the Asian communist countries of China, North Korea, and what was then North Vietnam, but most observers feel that severe undernutrition is probably rare in these societies. Some suggest that these latest U.N. estimates still overstate the problem, especially in the cases of Africa and the Near East. On the other hand, the study's authors claim that they used a quite restrictive notion of adequate nutrition and that "a less conservative definition might give a much higher figure" for the undernourished. Furthermore, the years of the survey—1969 through 1971—were years of generally good weather, high production, and low food prices. Large jumps in food prices nearly everywhere in subsequent years have undoubtedly pushed people who were formerly on the borders of undernutrition into that unhappy state.

Whatever the exact number, hundreds of millions of people are simply not getting enough food to lead fully active, healthy lives. Some in this group suffer from undernutrition so extreme that it threatens their existence directly. Community examinations show that at any given time about 1 to 7 percent of the pre-school children in poor countries weigh less than 60 percent of their expected weights—a desperate condition akin to walking death.[3] It is among this exceptionally deprived minority of children that the vicious, often fatal diseases of severe undernutrition are apt to appear: the protein-deficiency disease kwashiorkor, characterized by bloated bellies, wasted muscles, and apathy; and marasmus, which results from gross shortages of energy and protein and leaves its victims looking like little more than bags of bones and skin.

Severe undernutrition mainly strikes small children, who need about twice as much protein and energy in relation to overall body weight

"Even when undernutrition is not directly
lethal, it raises the odds of early death
from other causes."

as adults require. Pregnant and nursing mothers, who also need extra food, form a second nutritionally vulnerable group. Unfortunately, in many cultures a tradition of discriminating against small children and females of all ages in the allocation of family food supplies makes these two groups all the more vulnerable.

11

Available population studies show that the severely undernourished, those close to starvation, probably number in the tens rather than the hundreds of millions. While a far cry from the stereotypical notion that "half the world is starving to death," this number is still unconscionably large. When they do not starve, these victims of the modern economic order face the possibility of living with irreversibly stunted bodies and minds. And the clinical surveys also reveal that significant, if less dramatic, undernutrition affects as many as half to two-thirds of the children in the poor countries.[4] Even when undernutrition is not directly lethal, it raises the odds of early death from other causes. At the least, it impairs health and infringes upon the right to a full life.

In addition to energy and protein shortages, the problem of undernutrition encompasses numerous specific vitamin and mineral deficiencies that usually, but not always, coexist with overall underfeeding.[5] By far the most widespread of these is anemia, a condition often resulting from inadequate intake of iron or other vitamins, as well as from iron losses to blood parasites like hookworm. Widespread in rich and poor countries alike, anemia afflicts 5 to 15 percent of adult men and even higher proportions of women and children in many regions. Anemia saps the energy needed to work and raises susceptibility to disease; it also multiplies women's chances of dying during childbirth.

Deficiencies of vitamin A rank as the leading cause of childhood blindness in many developing countries. Xeropthalmia (literally, "dry eye") is the general term for ocular disorders brought on by vitamin A shortages, disorders that range from an inability to see in dim light to total blindness. A tenth of India's children are said to suffer "night blindness" as a result of this deficiency. Worldwide, probably between 20,000 and 100,000 children lose their sight completely every year for want of vitamin A.

Geographic comparisons of the scale of protein-calorie undernutrition are necessarily imprecise; the quality and kinds of information available vary considerably from one country to another. Nevertheless, available data show that a majority of the world's undernourished live in Asia. In the densely populated and desperately poor countries of the Indian subcontinent—in India, Pakistan, and Bangladesh—populations are especially hard-hit. There, more people live in destitution and on less land than in any other large region. Vast numbers of South Asians live on the edge of survival, staving off nutritional disaster only until the inevitable failure of the monsoon every several years. Unpublished dietary surveys in India commissioned by UNICEF in 1974 reveal the sorry dietary plight of a staggering number of human beings. Some 224 million of India's 600 million people consume less than three-fourths of the calories they need. Fifty-three million Indians take in less than half their minimum daily energy requirements.

A generation back, China also teemed with the undernourished and the outright starving. None of the hundreds of scientists, journalists, and doctors visiting China in the last few years, however, has reported observing any of the clinical signs of undernutrition that once blighted Chinese life.[6] Undernutrition in China has not been suppressed by dramatic national gains in per capita food production, but rather by more equitable distribution of available foods.

Africa has not yet reached the extremes of population density seen in parts of Asia such as Java or Bangladesh. But since extreme poverty is endemic, since modern agricultural techniques are rarely used, and since the farming potential of large areas is limited, undernutrition is widespread. The recent lengthy drought in the Sahelian zone, just south of the Sahara, shocked the world into recognizing the threat of periodic famine that imperils many Africans. Tens of millions of unnoticed others, however, also struggle against a chronic insufficiency of food. About 30 percent of sub-Saharan Africa's children, calculates the World Health Organization (WHO), are not consuming the nutrients they need. Another 4 percent suffer severe, life-threatening undernutrition.[7]

Average incomes throughout most of Latin America are considerably higher than those in most of Asia and Africa. Drastic disparities in income and access to farmland, however, have given undernutrition a long leash among the poor. According to the Pan American Health Organization (PAHO), from about 10 to 30 percent of the children in most Latin American countries suffer at least moderate degrees of undernutrition. Nutritional deficiencies are most widespread in places such as Northeast Brazil, the Andes Mountains, and parts of Central America and the Caribbean, where economic exploitation and poverty are the harshest. Haiti, with its deadly trinity of extreme population density, ecological devastation, and exceptional income disparity, has one of the world's highest rates of severe undernutrition among children—7 percent.[8]

13

Oddly enough, little more is known about the prevalence of undernutrition in many rich countries than is known about its presence in the poor countries. In wealthy nations, generally high incomes and more or less adequate social welfare programs prevent much of the serious protein-calorie malnutrition of the sort rampant in the developing nations. Yet even in a country as rich as the United States, millions of people live in dire need and some live so far outside the mainstream of national life that government aid programs such as the food stamp program never reach them.

One basic question is left unanswered by available surveys of the nutritional state of Americans: How many are undernourished? Current investigations reveal that mineral and vitamin deficiencies are widespread among the populace. But studies over the last decade have proved that more serious undernutrition does plague the American poor, especially minority ethnic groups, Indians living on reservations, migrant workers, and the aged.[9] Well-publicized journeys by national political leaders into zones of deep poverty in the late 1960s exposed the entire nation to people with the vacant stares and underdeveloped bodies that are a common legacy of the undernourished poor everywhere. Those forays showed that even in a country where obesity is the leading nutritional disorder, economic deprivation can exact its customary nutritional cost.

Undernutrition and Disease

Deaths overtly due to underconsumption are uncommon. But the far broader and more insidious effects of nutritional deficiencies on human well-being are not. Simply put, deficient diets increase the likelihood and worsen the consequences of many other health threats. Inadequate or improper food supplies are now strongly implicated as the principal cause of the inordinately high mortality in the poor countries.[10]

Undernutrition hits small children hardest; their high death rate in the developing countries is the chief distinguishing factor between the state of health there and that in the more developed world. In many of the poorer countries, two-thirds of all deaths occur among children under five.

By far the most extensive and reliable investigation of childhood mortality in the developing world is that published by PAHO in 1973, which examined deaths among young children in 15 varied regions in the Americas.[11] This study showed either nutritional deficiencies or infant immaturity at birth to be the *primary* cause of only 6 percent of deaths among children under five (immaturity includes both premature births and underweight births regardless of timing, and is often associated with poor nutrition among mothers). However, nutritional deficiencies and immaturity were found to be *associated* with 57 percent of all child deaths. Undernutrition thus probably contributes to more than half of all child deaths in Latin America; a comparable calculation in South Asia or Central Africa would likely yield an even higher figure.

As the numerous deaths associated with immature births imply, undernutrition can injure even an unborn child. Underweight or premature births stem, of course, from various causes, and such births are often associated with infant deaths even when nutrition is adequate. Underweight babies are especially susceptible to infections, and this frailty sometimes persists well beyond their earliest days of life. The exact impact of maternal nutrition on birth weights has not been well established, but evidence suggests that the influence begins long before a child is even conceived. In fact, the childhood diet of the mother, which helped determine her physical size and overall health, usually affects the newborn's size. When a mother has been undernourished and unhealthy during her childhood, writes a prominent physician, "her pregnancy is more frequently disturbed and her child more often of low birth-weight."[12] Thus undernutrition among girls today imperils the health of the next generation.

Less surprisingly, studies have also revealed that the infant, as well as the mother, can be harmed by dietary deficiencies *during* the mother's pregnancy, especially when the mother has a history of undernutrition. Nutritionists in Guatemala who provided food supplements to pregnant women in two villages found that the average birth weights of babies born to the women increased by 9 percent over the pre-study average. A research group working in another Guatemalan village discovered that "contrary to the belief that the developing infant could successfully parasitize the mother for whatever nutrients were needed for growth, . . . newborns in the village are not normal—they are small at birth . . . and nearly 20 percent show evidence of subtle intrauterine infection."[13]

15

Of all deaths among children under age five covered in the PAHO study, nearly four-fifths occurred during the victim's first year of life. The riskiest day for the newborn is the first, and it is in the earliest days of life that the threats associated with underweight birth hold most force. Then, in the following months and years, the baleful synergism of infection and malnutrition takes hold wherever conditions allow.

Limited and impure water supplies, inadequate sanitary facilities and habits, and substandard housing together expose youngsters in developing countries to a host of infectious agents. Forty-five newborns in Guatemala who were studied during the first three years of their lives suffered a total of nearly 2,500 episodes of infectious disease during that brief period—an average of one disease every three weeks per infant.[14] Weakened by poor nutrition, children living in unsanitary conditions succumb to the infectious agents ubiquitous in their environment much more often than they would if they were properly fed. And when they do fall ill, the undernourished are far more likely than better-fed children to suffer severely. Diseases considered "routine" in more developed regions—diarrhea, measles, or chicken pox—are a routine cause of death among the poor.

Before the recent large-scale use of vaccine in many countries, measles afflicted children virtually everywhere. Yet, while fatalities from measles have long been rare in developed countries, death rates among those contracting measles in poor regions are sometimes as high as 15 percent. In some years, the fatality rate among children infected with measles in Mexico is 180 times higher than that in the United States, and the fatality rate in Ecuador is 480 times higher. Neither a variation in the virulence of measles viruses in different countries nor variations in human immunity to the disease explains these differences; all evidence indicts nutritional factors as the primary cause of these radical disparities in the disease's impact. International comparisons of death rates from several other infections—among them whooping cough, tuberculosis, and diarrhea—reveal similar disparities.[15]

Just as undernutrition aggravates disease, infections may, conversely, cause nutritional stress in those whose diets would otherwise be barely adequate. Infections in the gastrointestinal tract reduce the body's ability to extract nutrients from food, and, even more significant, nearly all infections trigger an increased elimination of protein nitrogen through body wastes. Moreover, well-meaning parents often put children with gastrointestinal problems on diets less nutritious than usual in accordance with local notions about which foods are appropriate for the sick. Well-fed children can easily replace the nutrients lost and tissues damaged by infection, but those living on the margins of malnutrition may never make up the deficit.

Most deaths associated with infant undernutrition occur during or after weaning, as mother's milk is supplemented with or replaced by other foods. The foods substituted for mother's milk during this critical period frequently fail to meet the child's nutritional needs, and the introduction of new foods in an unsanitary milieu exposes the child to a multitude of infectious agents. As leading nutritionists Nevin Scrimshaw and Moisés Béhar observe, the mortality rate of children from one to four years of age—those in the postweaning period—is the best measure of malnutrition in a country.[16] In more developed regions, only about one death occurs per thousand children aged one to four. In some of the poorest areas, forty or fifty deaths per thousand children occur—most of them preventable through better diets.

The interacting threats associated with weaning, undernutrition, and poor sanitation are illustrated most forcefully by the problem of diar-

"The mortality rate of children from one to four years of age is the best measure of malnutrition in a country."

rhea. Those in well-nourished countries, for whom diarrhea is usually no more than an occasional nuisance brought on by impure food or forays into a foreign cuisine, may be surprised to learn that, worldwide, diarrhea is a major killer. The upper respiratory infections known as the common cold cause more discomfort than any other known disease, but diarrhea outranks them as a cause of death.

17

Diarrhea takes children's lives in all countries, but its death toll today is small in affluent areas. In contrast, in many poorer countries, deaths from diarrhea (concentrated among children) outnumber those from any other cause in the entire population. There is nothing historically unique about this dismal picture. At the beginning of the current century, children in Western Europe and North America succumbed to diarrhea at rates even higher than those of the poorest countries today. But improved diets and sanitation have left their mark, pushing down diarrhea-caused death rates for young children in these areas by a factor of more than a hundred.[17]

Stressing the vulnerability of the young child, physicians have adopted the term "weanling diarrhea" to describe this deleterious syndrome. The name itself evokes the mutually reinforcing nature of infection and undernutrition. Diarrhea may strike a child any time after birth and is especially common in infants born underweight, but its frequency escalates radically during the weaning period, usually after the age of six months. As food supplements to breast feeding become necessary, exposure to unsterile foods and containers is inevitable, and an increasingly mobile infant is an increasingly exposed infant. Few babies between the ages of six months and two years in developing countries escape diarrhea, and many suffer repeated episodes.

The trend toward premature abandonment of breast feeding in the swelling cities of Africa, Asia, and Latin America is boosting the frequency and severity of weanling diarrhea. Bottle feeding in an unsanitary milieu raises the odds of exposure to infection and, when parents cannot afford proper substitutes for nutritious breast milk, subsequent malnutrition lowers infant resistance to disease.[18]

Unsanitary living conditions and personal habits also promote weanling diarrhea. The bacteria and viruses that apparently cause diarrhea are passed from person to person through fecally contaminated food, water, and utensils, or, perhaps most often, from hand to mouth. Studies of diarrheal diseases have concluded that convenient access to adequate quantities of water, even water of less than perfect quality, is of utmost importance to efforts to control the disease. Personal cleanliness, the indispensable control measure, is impossible where the only available water must be head-carried several kilometers by women and children.

Sanitary conditions determine its frequency, but nutrition, more than any other factor, influences the severity of diarrhea. Among the better-off, diarrhea usually causes a few days of mild discomfort. In an environment of poverty, the disease's acute phase commonly lasts four to five days and usually entails a fever. Among poorly nourished children, report the authors of a WHO study, "a low-grade indisposition often continues for a month or more, sometimes as long as three months, with irregularly recurring loose stools, a progressively depleted nutritional state, and occasional recurrent acute episodes."[19] Some undernourished children suffer chronically recurring diarrhea for years.

In poor regions, one to four of every hundred children under the age of two who contracts diarrhea dies from it. The PAHO studies in Latin America revealed that, in many areas, diarrhea caused a third or more of all deaths among those under five. In three Guatemalan villages studied in the 1950s, diarrhea accounted for 27 percent of all deaths in the *general* population, its toll especially great among small children. Yet, as surviving children gradually become acclimated to the disease agents prevalent in their local environment, their resistance increases. For many reasons, older children are also more likely to be adequately fed. Thus, both the frequency of diarrhea and its death toll fall as children grow older.

As this brief review implies, the measure of undernutrition's toll must be taken in the total environment in which it occurs. Apart from diseases clearly linked to particular dietary deficiencies, undernutrition abets other disease agents surely and insidiously. Good health requires the elimination of both nutritional stress and other environmental sources of illness. Even the most modern medical practices will be severely undermined where undernutrition is rampant.

Malnourished Minds

Premature death is the cruelest sacrifice exacted by a social order that sanctions undernutrition. But other costs—also dreadful, if less absolute—are borne by those surviving the combined ravages of poor diets and disease. Severe undernutrition in early childhood, a growing body of evidence indicates, can stunt a child's physical and intellectual development. Combined with the social deprivations of poverty, undernutrition can impair reasoning powers, language and motor skills, and social behavior, thereby denying individuals the basic right to realize the human potential carried in their genes. If a child is underfed long enough during a critical period of development, no amount of compensatory feeding or education can fully restore what has been lost.

Though widely acknowledged by nutritionists and pediatricians, undernutrition's potential to inflict lasting personal damage may never be unequivocally proven by usual scientific means and standards. The awesome complexities of the human mind, and of personality formation, assure uncertainty. Although direct nutritional effects on the brain and nervous system are physical, the activity of thinking—however grounded in physical processes—involves impalpable acts of creation. To demonstrate an alteration in the number or size of certain brain cells is not necessarily to predict the resulting intellectual and behavioral consequences.

The human brain does not mature by bread alone. Severe undernutrition virtually always occurs in a deprived social environment that can itself stunt intellectual development. Undernourished children are more apt than the well-fed to live in serious poverty, to suffer frequent illness, to have parents who are illiterate or who did poorly in school, and to be deprived of the enriching experiences that stimulate intellectual development. A lack of stimulation results in more than a gap in accumulated knowledge; it can, like nutritional deficiencies, actually influence the brain's physical development.

Studies of humans and animals have established unequivocally that severe malnutrition early in life decreases the size of the brain and alters its cellular composition. What remains uncertain is the subsequent influence these changes have on learning and behavior. Numerous studies of humans have clearly proven an association between severe early undernutrition and impaired learning abilities. Because of the concerns just noted, categorical claims of *causation* cannot be made, but available evidence points strongly toward childhood undernutrition as one contributor to lifetime intellectual deficiencies. Following an exhaustive review of the research literature, a committee of the U.S. National Academy of Sciences has concluded that "the weight of evidence seems to indicate that early and severe malnutrition is an important factor in later intellectual development, above and beyond the effects of social-familial influences."[20]

An elaborate study in a Mexican village, for example, established that children who had recovered from severe undernutrition lagged behind others in the development of language skills and in the ability to form concepts. Comparisons of stimulation in the home environment failed to explain the differences fully. Another study in Chile compared the intellectual performances of children malnourished in infancy to those of children who had been well-fed. Though the two groups came from environments that were apparently almost identical in other respects, the formerly malnourished scored notably lower on intelligence tests than did their well-fed counterparts.[21]

In 1964, researchers in Indonesia tested some five to twelve-year-old children whose nutritional status in the late fifties had been recorded in another study. All the 117 children under study were from the same low socio-economic class. The investigators found that the children's intellectual as well as physical development could be predicted fairly accurately on the basis of their nutritional status during the preschool years. Previously malnourished children who had shown clinical signs of vitamin A deficiency between the ages of two and four had the lowest scores on intelligence tests, while those who had never been diagnosed as malnourished had the highest scores.[22]

The likelihood that such learning disabilities are in some measure irreversible emerges forbodingly from findings on the timing and nature of brain development. Like the rest of the body, the brain and its critical message systems do not grow uniformly throughout life; instead, most maturation takes place during a period of rapid development called the growth spurt. But the brain's growth spurt is far shorter than that of the rest of the body. At birth the human brain has already reached 25 percent of its adult weight, and after one year it weighs 70 percent of its adult potential. In contrast, overall body weight at birth is usually about 5 percent of that at maturity, and even at age ten, most people weigh only about half their adult total.

21

A particularly crucial attribute of the brain's growth spurt, which probably lasts from about the twentieth week of fetal life to two years after birth, is its apparent chronological inflexibility. The body seems to obey some inviolable time regulations; if certain kinds of growth do not occur within the specified period, the opportunity for that growth may be lost forever.[23] The period presents a once-in-a-lifetime opportunity for normal development, which is why undernutrition among pregnant women and small children has implications profoundly graver than those of undernutrition among any other group.

Fortunately, the wondrous complexity of human intellectual development demands qualifications about the impact of nutritional deficiencies even in the initial years of life. A recent study of Korean children who were adopted by U.S. parents underscores the potential of an exceptionally supportive social environment to mitigate the intellectual legacy of undernutrition.

Those Korean-American school children who had shown signs of malnutrition when adopted (at an average age of 18 months) now score as well on intelligence tests, and perform as well in the classroom, as the average U.S. child. On the other hand, those adopted Korean children who were well-fed in infancy score and perform *better* than the average child in the United States. Thus the formerly malnourished still lag behind those with a comparable home environment.[24]

Virtually all research on the intellectual impact of dietary deficiencies has focused on people suffering from severe protein-calorie malnutrition. Children once hospitalized with identifiable acute conditions such as marasmus or kwashiorkor are most often studied. Yet for every child who is severely undernourished, many more suffer milder, chronic dietary deficiencies. To determine whether or not moderate undernutrition can also cause lasting intellectual damage is to describe the fate of untold numbers of children.

Clearly, moderate undernutrition and a deficient social environment together impair a child's later intellectual performance, but the relative contributions of each factor are little understood. The U.S. National Academy of Sciences has declared that studies relating "moderate malnutrition . . . to later intellectual performance have frequently found that malnutrition does play a role apart from factors related to social status. This is a tentative conclusion, however, and confirmation awaits more systematic research." Support for this position comes from studies of animal brain development. Some tests have revealed incomplete development of the cerebral cortex in animals suffering even moderate undernutrition throughout critical periods in early life.[25]

The debate over the exact roles of early undernutrition and social deprivation in impairing learning abilities is largely academic. The two negative forces virtually always coexist, reinforcing each other. Moreover, apart from possible harm to the brain and nervous system, undernutrition can impair intellectual potential through its indirect impact on personality formation. Undernutrition accentuates—and even creates—the other environmental deprivations of stimulation and experience that hinder personal development. Often apathetic and socially withdrawn, the poorly nourished tend to be less socially interactive than the well-fed. Physical and mental fatigue, the inability to concentrate, and low motivation all doom them to poor performance at school; and frequent illness means frequent absence from the classroom. Thus the poorly nourished child falls behind in a critical learning period, suffering what Alan Berg has called "an irreversible loss of opportunity," whether or not his brain has been physically damaged.[26]

Perhaps the chief lesson of the still incomplete research record on nutrition and learning is that undernutrition, disease, and poverty are deeply interwoven. Good nutrition alone will not prevent or erase the scars of poverty, and, in the face of undernutrition, even the most creative educational efforts may fail. Our knowledge of human brain development imparts a special urgency to efforts to provide an adequate diet to pregnant and nursing mothers, and to children un-

"The refined meat-heavy diet is also
enticing the well-heeled urban elite in
Africa, Asia, and Latin America."

der two years old. At the same time, ample evidence shows that improved diets and social conditions at any stage of life benefit the individual.

The Emergence of the Affluent Diet   23

The stamp of each culture's cuisine is unique; the Americans have hamburgers, the French rich sauces, the Japanese raw fish. Nevertheless, when the basic nutritional components rather than the particular dishes of diets are analyzed, some pronounced international trends appear. One of the most conspicuous trends to emerge over the last century or so is a consumption pattern in the industrial Western countries that is sometimes called the "affluent diet."

The affluent diet flourishes only where incomes range far above subsistence level and where people have market access to a highly productive agricultural system—hence its name. Those with an affluent diet consume large amounts of animal proteins and fats in the forms of meats and dairy products; they substitute highly refined flour and sugar for bulky carbohydrates like whole grains, tubers, fruits, and vegetables; and, increasingly, they choose commercially manufactured foods over fresh, unprocessed products. Never before the present century have large numbers of people maintained such a diet.

The affluent diet is most deeply entrenched in North America, but it has taken hold in Western Europe too. Japan and the Soviet Union, late starters in the transition away from traditional grain or potato-centered diets, are quickly making up for lost time. The "refined" meat-heavy diet is also enticing the well-heeled urban elite in Africa, Asia, and Latin America. At the marketplace and at the dinner table, people are proving that the appeals of meat, refined flour, and sugar transcend borders and cultural conventions.

By the traditional measures of good nutrition, the affluent diet should be a healthy one. Protein supplies are generous; energy intake is adequate, though sometimes excessive; and key vitamin and mineral requirements are met. Viewed against the backdrop of humanity's long history of nutrient-deficiency diseases such as scurvy and pellagra, and of rampant present-day undernutrition, the affluent diet looks healthy indeed.

But nutritional appearances can deceive. Observed links between the way people in the industrial countries eat and the way they live and die have raised new questions about the soundness of the affluent diet. Such connections have forced nutritionists and doctors to view this diet from new angles, and to refigure the meaning of "good nutrition." They have also forced experts to evaluate a given diet within the context of a particular lifestyle. The conclusions springing from this reassessment are sobering, if not startling: like most "get rich quick" schemes, the quest for rich foods entails grave risks.

The most suspect characteristics of the affluent diet are its high levels of fats, especially animal fats, and cholesterol. Most people know that greasy fried foods, butter, and salad oil contain fats; fewer realize that much of our fat intake comes in less obvious forms. Meats, especially beef and pork (which contain more fat than do poultry and fish), as well as dairy products and vegetable oils, all add fat to the diet. Cholesterol, highly publicized because it has been associated with circulatory ailments, is most concentrated in eggs and liver. But it is also present in other animal products.

In the Western countries, fats have accounted for an increasing proportion of total caloric intake over the last century. Largely because they eat more meat and dairy products, people in the industrial countries consume far more fat than those, such as the Greeks, whose cuisines are visibly oil-laden. Fats sometimes account for 45 to 50 percent of the calories in a North American's diet; the national average is over 40 percent in many Western countries. In contrast, fats comprise less than a fourth of the food energy consumed in most poor countries.

The quantity of fat that people eat probably matters less than the kind of fat they eat. In particular, a high intake of saturated fats, those supplied mainly but not entirely by animal products, is thought to promote cardiovascular problems and, possibly, various forms of cancer. Unsaturated fats, plentiful in most animal and vegetable fat sources, seem to entail fewer health risks.

Opposing forces have influenced the relative intake of vegetable and animal fats in developed countries. Economic and health considerations have moved people to shift from butter to vegetable-based margarines, and from lard to hydrogenated vegetable oils. At the same time, climbing meat consumption has partly offset the health benefits of that shift; animal-fat intake has remained high and total fat consumption has been driven upward.

Average consumption of meats, including poultry, in the United States, Australia, and Argentina has now leveled off at close to 250 pounds (carcass weight) a year per capita. Citizens of France, West Germany, and Canada now each consume close to 200 pounds a year, while those in other European countries eat smaller but generally increasing amounts of meat. Among the richer countries, Japan lags conspicuously behind in meat consumption, but its per capita intake of 44 pounds in 1974 represented a spectacular 428 percent jump over the 1961 level. In contrast, average meat consumption in many low-income countries ranges below 20 pounds a year.

High in fats, the affluent diet is also low in whole grains. Ironically, *total* grain use in the developed countries has risen markedly over recent decades. At between one and two thousand pounds per capita, consumption is now two to five times that in poorer countries. But an increasing share of this grain is consumed indirectly, as meat from grain-fed animals. Thus we forfeit the possible benefits of whole grains to animals only to lard our diets. "Prime" beef, the highly marbled type for which consumers pay premium prices, exemplifies this changeover perfectly. Prime beef is produced by raising cattle on feedlots, where they consume about ten pounds of grain for every pound of meat added during their stay. Since grain-fed beef contains more fat than does range-fed beef, people pay extra for a product that, at current consumption levels in many countries, is more likely than less fatty meats to threaten their well-being.

Not only is direct grain consumption low in the affluent diet, but most of the fiber, or roughage, present in the outer layers of grain has also disappeared. In rich nations, wheat is usually milled into refined white flour. Raw or lightly cooked fruits and vegetables, which also provide roughage, are increasingly being passed over in favor of canned or frozen foods, which are often overcooked. Even the fruits and vegetables that are bought fresh are often peeled or over-cooked. Unfortunately, reducing dietary roughage apparently alters the chemistry of digestion and the physical properties of body wastes, in turn possibly promoting a host of diseases of the digestive system.

Starch intake has dropped precipitously along with the consumption of bulky foods and fiber in the affluent diet, only to be replaced by the dental scourge, refined sugar. In fact, global per capita sugar consumption has grown by half just since 1950, and the average person in the world now eats 44 pounds of sugar a year. Health problems other than tooth decay—painful and expensive as that is—have apparently grown along with the world's sweet tooth; high sugar intake is linked by many to diabetes and other diseases. Most traditional societies don't use refined sugar at all, and recipes calling for sugar were rare in Europe and North America a few centuries back. Today, high sugar consumption plagues all the developed and many of the less developed countries. Whether consumed in candy and soft drinks or in baked goods and manufactured foods, sugar has found a following. Cubans, Costa Ricans, Americans, Australians, and Israelis each down over a hundred pounds of sugar a year, while Western Europeans eat an average of 90 pounds each. By contrast, annual sugar consumption in Japan, Taiwan, and the Philippines, though climbing fast, is only about 50 pounds per person; and sugar intake in many poor countries is much lower still.

As the affluent diet has spread, so have a wide variety of heretofore rare diseases such as coronary heart disease, diabetes, diverticulosis, and bowel cancer. Confined largely to those leading the lifestyles of the developed Western world, whether in Paris or Singapore, these ailments are sometimes collectively called the "diseases of civilization." Where these diseases of the privileged prevail, improved sanitation and ample food supplies have largely stamped out fatal infections and undernutrition—which have been replaced by modern ailments that strike the young and middle-aged as well as the old. Some ingredients of modern Western life—and dietary factors are among the leading suspects—are abetting these killers.

Medical detectives are slowly unravelling the intricate web of interconnections that link the affluent diet to the various diseases of civili-

"Recipes calling for sugar were rare in
Europe and North America a few centuries
back."

zation. Combined with a sedentary lifestyle, high calorie consumption
leads to obesity, which in turn encourages diabetes, hypertension,
and coronary heart disease. High intake of refined foods such as
sugar and flour may encourage diverticulosis and a host of other
conditions, while high salt intake facilitates the development of hypertension. Diabetes and hypertension, killers themselves, also
greatly boost the risk of coronary heart disease and, in the case of hypertension, stroke. A diet high in animal fats fosters arterial problems
that can lead to a coronary attack or stroke. Finally, fats may also
be linked to the genesis of bowel, breast, prostate, and other types
of cancer.

27

Both affluent diets and sedentary lifestyles represent radical depar-
tures from the conditions under which humans evolved for millions
of years. That our bodies should rebel is hardly surprising.

A Modern Epidemic: Coronary Heart Disease

Seldom has one disease so dominated an era. Coronary heart disease,
once a rare affliction even among the aged, is now the leading killer
of the old and the middle-aged in many countries; and it sometimes
takes the lives of the young as well. The affluent diet and sedentary
lifestyles are contributing to this trend, not only in the developed
world, but also in the cities of the poor countries, where coronary
heart disease is emerging as an important health problem.

All cardiovascular diseases together, including coronary and other
heart diseases, strokes, arterial diseases, and others, account for
about *one-half* of all deaths in the industrialized countries. Coronary
heart disease, which involves the coronary arteries through which
the heart supplies itself with blood, often culminates in a "heart attack" when the blood supply is cut off. This disease accounts for one
in every three deaths in the United States, claiming annually some
700,000 lives. In Japan and France, cerebrovascular disease, or stroke,
which involves an impaired supply of blood to parts of the brain,
takes even more lives than does coronary heart disease.

World Health Organization data for 18 Western countries reveal increases in the incidence of coronary heart disease between 1950 and
1968 for every age group. Among those aged 35-44, the incidence

rose by more than 50 percent, and, among those aged 45-54, by more than 30 percent. In the United States, where coronary heart disease fatalities are more prevalent than in any other large country, the frequency of deaths from this disease for most age groups has tapered off somewhat since the early 1960s. Both changing lifestyles and improved medical treatment of heart-disease victims have probably contributed to this downturn. In the United Kingdom, too, the death rate among men from coronary heart disease has stopped rising since 1965. But incidence rates are still climbing almost everywhere else.[27]

In India, what sketchy information exists shows that the number of coronary heart disease patients in urban hospitals has been increasing steadily over the past 20 years. The incidence of coronary heart disease is on the rise in China as well. According to a WHO report, coronary heart disease, though still limited, occurs more and more frequently in Sri Lanka, Korea, Malaysia, and the Philippines, especially among people under 40.[28]

Doctors at the Bir hospital in Kathmandu, Nepal, have noted that the annual number of heart attacks increased from three to thirty between 1960 and 1973—an insignificant number, perhaps, by Western standards but enough to suggest that the changing lifestyle in the capital has had an influence. In the Ivory Coast, physicians have noted the emergence of coronary heart disease among the more affluent classes of Abidjan. One study of these urban heart disease patients found that nine of every ten victims were male and that their average age was only 53. In 17 out of 22 countries in North and South America, the disease is now one of the five principal causes of death. In ten of these countries, heart disease is the number one killer.[29]

In Japan, coronary disease rates have tripled over the last 15 years. Yet the annual coronary death toll is still low compared to the toll from stroke, which accounts for one of every four deaths among those aged 75 or under.[30] Compared to Europeans and Americans, the Japanese consume relatively little animal fat, and this dietary preference seems partially to protect them from coronary disease.

Populations that eat large quantities of animal fat tend to have higher coronary death rates than those populations that consume smaller quantities of animal fat. Yet high saturated-fat consumption is only one of the "risk factors" that have been associated with coronary disease. Obesity, high blood cholesterol, diabetes, hypertension, sedentary living, stress, and cigarette smoking can all raise the risk of coronary disease. Males, heavy drinkers, those with a family history of the disease, and those who drink soft (mineral-free) water also run higher-than-normal risks.

In discussing traits that are associated with an increased risk of heart disease, doctors use the term "risk factor" rather than the term "cause." They do so in part because few cause-and-effect relationships have been absolutely established in this area of inquiry, and in part because no single "cause" can usually be held accountable for the present epidemic of degenerative diseases.

The noted Framingham study examined the interrelationship between the risk of developing coronary heart disease and such factors as weight change, cholesterol in the blood, and blood-pressure levels. For 12 years doctors examined more than 5,000 men and women over the age of 30 in Framingham, Massachusetts, for the initial development of coronary disease. Angina pectoris, or chest pain, which is frequently an early indicator of coronary disease, was more common among obese men both with and without elevated blood pressure and blood cholesterol. Yet for women, obesity did not increase the chances of angina unless accompanied by high blood pressure and high blood cholesterol.

The greater the number of risk factors present in a person's life, the greater the danger. A 45-year-old American man who smokes more than a pack of cigarettes a day doubles his odds of a heart attack. But the 45-year-old smoker with high blood pressure and a high blood-cholesterol level runs nearly *four times* the risk of a heart attack as does a man who is subject to none of these factors.[31]

Socio-economic levels also seem to correlate with the incidence of coronary heart disease. As median family incomes rise, death rates from coronary heart disease drop. Upper-middle and middle classes in the United States suffer from proportionately less coronary disease than they did before World War II, and both have lower coronary death rates than the poor.

Apparently, the rich in the United States are now more aware of the various risk factors associated with heart attacks than are the poor, and have adjusted their lifestyles accordingly. But those in the lower economic classes have rushed to embrace the same affluent diets and sedentary lifestyles that were once the exclusive privileges of the wealthy. Whether other countries now raising their living standards will follow the full cycle of rising and falling heart disease rates experienced by the United States is an open question. Many premature coronary deaths in developing countries could probably be avoided, however, if public health authorities would establish programs designed to help people avoid the known risk factors.

Genetic factors influence the development of coronary heart disease, but their role is still not well understood. In Finland, the difference in coronary mortality rates between the eastern and western parts of the country is apparently partly genetic in origin. Finns from the east have thicker inner layers in their coronary arteries than do their counterparts in western Finland. Genetically predisposed to the early onset of atherosclerosis and raised on a diet extremely high in animal fats, adults from the east have one of the world's highest coronary death rates.[32]

People born with the "familial type II" gene are especially liable to develop heart disease. As many as one in 200 newborns in the United States may harbor this deadly trait, and perhaps four out of five male babies so affected will develop coronary heart disease by the age of 60. More males than females inherit this gene, a fact that partially explains males' higher susceptibility to coronary heart disease. Female sex hormones also seem to provide women with some protection from atherosclerosis and heart attacks. During the 12-year Framingham study, 252 men and only 128 women developed coronary heart disease, and the men developed much more serious forms of the disease than did the women. Female coronary heart disease rates are affected by lifestyle and diet, just as male rates are, but the gap in death rates between the two sexes is nevertheless large.[33]

Atherosclerosis, the partial blockage of arteries with tissue growth and fatty deposits, leads to coronary heart disease when the coronary arteries are affected. Since these arteries supply blood directly to the heart, a heart attack will result if they become sufficiently clogged.

Any population suffering from a high incidence of atherosclerosis will almost certainly have high coronary heart disease rates as well.

The accumulation of deposits in the arteries seems to be affected by the consumption of saturated fats and cholesterol. These food components appear to contribute to the chain of events that leads from a high cholesterol blood-count to atherosclerosis, and, finally, to a completely blocked coronary artery and a heart attack. Just what determines the level of cholesterol in the blood and how a high blood-cholesterol level is translated into atherosclerosis are as yet unanswered questions. But considerable evidence shows that a diet high in unsaturated fats lowers the cholesterol output of the body, while high intake of saturated fats, such as those in meat and dairy products, apparently stimulates the liver to produce more cholesterol.

High consumption of meat, eggs, and other cholesterol-rich foods can raise cholesterol levels in the blood stream by about 10 percent. Other factors such as weight, exercise, and heredity also affect the body's cholesterol production. The Food and Nutrition Board of the U.S. National Academy of Sciences has declared that there is "abundant evidence that the risk of developing coronary heart disease is positively correlated with the level of cholesterol in the (blood) plasma . . . and that the level of cholesterol can be lowered by appropriate dietary modifications."[34]

In the nineteenth century, an apparent association between the stressful lives of doctors and their relatively high susceptibility to heart attacks was noticed. In fact, the occasional cases of coronary heart disease were known as the "doctors' disease." Some researchers today also contend that coronary heart disease and the combined effects of a high-fat diet and competitive, stressful living go hand in hand.

The body reacts to stress by releasing various hormones into the blood stream. These hormones seem, in turn, to affect the way the body breaks down fats and cholesterol. Diet apparently alters the effects of stress on blood cholesterol. According to one heart specialist, "The potential for harm to the cardiovascular system by stressful patterns of living is markedly diminished if not nullified by subsistence on a diet low in fat. A low incidence of coronary heart disease reported for racial groups in 'low-fat,' 'high-stress' countries such as China, Japan, Korea, and Yemen must lead to such a conclusion."[35]

32 In the rich countries, signs of atherosclerosis now appear in teenagers as well as in the middle-aged. Thus measures aimed at preventing atherosclerosis should be introduced early in life and must be long-lasting. While researchers have yet to prove that exercise retards or stops arterial clogging, some authorities believe that it can, and they think that regular exercise reduces the likelihood and damage of coronary heart disease. A recent U.S. study on the effect of diet and exercise on cholesterol levels in the blood showed that regular exercise in conjunction with a controlled-fat diet helped to reduce blood cholesterol and to maintain it at a low level. Regular exercise also increases the supply of oxygen to the muscles and makes the heart work more economically, perhaps thereby lowering a person's odds of suffering a heart attack. A 1974 report on diet and coronary heart disease by the Department of Health and Social Security in the United Kingdom identified lack of exercise as a risk factor equal in importance to high blood pressure, cigarette smoking, or high consumption of fats and sugar.[36]

The American Medical Association and medical authorities in Sweden, Norway, and the United Kingdom all exhort adults to reduce fat consumption. In their view, fats should supply less than 35 percent of total calories, as opposed to the 40-45 percent now common in these countries. Furthermore, according to the American Heart Association and others, most adult males should sharply reduce their intake of cholesterol. The daily level should not exceed 300 milligrams.[37] (One egg contains 250 mgs. of cholesterol, while a three ounce cooked piece of beef, pork, or chicken contains approximately 85 mgs.)

No diet and no amount of exercise can eliminate coronary heart disease. Elderly people, as well as some younger people who are genetically predisposed to the disease, will continue to die of heart attacks. However, hundreds of thousands of deaths each year from coronary heart disease are premature and avoidable. In North America and Europe, 10 percent of all coronary deaths strike those under the age of 55, and over half involve people under the age of 75. Most of these

could probably be prevented and could certainly be postponed by
changes in diet and lifestyle.

Homo Sedentarius and Obesity

33

Human beings long depended upon their legs for transportation
and upon their physical strength for the cultivation of food.
The overwhelming majority of people consumed barely enough to
survive while the privileged few ate rich, fattening diets. Re-
stricted to the elite, obesity came to be regarded as a status
symbol. The Roman senator's girth won him great prestige among
the mass of underfed plebeians, and Aga Khan's yearly weighings
were legendary among his people. Today in many of the less developed countries of the world the same attitudes still prevail.
In Nepal, for example, obesity is a mark of distinction, and the
present King would find it highly impolitic to go on a reducing
diet.

In North America, Japan, many European countries, and in other
developed nations around the world, the food supply is now more
abundant than ever before. Most people from all social classes can
get more than enough to eat; and with the emergence of the affluent diet, obesity is no longer the "privilege" of the elite.
In fact, excessive fat has become the scourge of the lower class
and, to the many Westerners who prize leanness, a mark of social dis-
dain. "Doppelkinnepidemie," the double-chin epidemic, has blos-
somed in West Germany since the postwar economic miracle. In the
United States, 10 to 20 percent of all children and 35 to 50 percent
of the middle-aged are overweight.

The increased prevalence of obesity is not, however, solely a function
of changing food supplies and of mercurial attitudes about the ideal
weight. Combined with individual genetic susceptibility to obesity,
two factors—caloric intake and expenditure of energy through physical activity—determine weight gains. In some rich countries calorie
consumption has actually fallen since the turn of the century, but not
as rapidly as the rate at which people exercise has declined. The after-
math of the Industrial Revolution, the age of the automobile and
household appliances, has changed the way people live. Fewer
and fewer jobs require physical work of any sort. Even the modern

farmer, perched atop his tractor, can be overweight and out of condition. Millions of office workers get no exercise whatever, save a short walk or an occasional sprint to catch the rush-hour bus. Ours is a sedentary civilization, and the species of *Homo sedentarius* has migrated from the cities and the suburbs to the countryside. Examining the food consumption and exercise patterns of Americans, nutritionist Jean Mayer found that

> Although our population has grown taller, we have grown heavier (and fatter) even faster—despite a slowly decreasing overall food intake. Clearly, the increased mechanization of our lives has diminished the level of physical activity much more rapidly than our caloric intake has dropped.[38]

Obesity, often defined as the condition of being 20 percent or more over a desirable weight determined mainly on the basis of health statistics, is not randomly distributed throughout society. Rather, in developed countries, the condition seems to be concentrated in the lowest socio-economic groups. A study performed in New York City showed that one of every three lower-class women was obese, compared to one in twenty among upper-class women. Obesity is more common among lower-class six-year-olds than among their upper-class counterparts.[39]

Obesity is more than a social problem; it interests the medical profession because obese people run a higher risk of premature death than do people of normal or below-normal weight. For example, men who are 10 percent overweight have a one-third greater chance of dying prematurely from ailments such as coronary heart disease, high blood pressure, and diabetes than do those of average weight. Men more than 20 percent overweight are one and a half times as likely to die prematurely. In recent testimony before the U.S. Senate, Dr. Theodore Cooper, Assistant Secretary of Health, Education, and Welfare, estimated that one-fifth of all Americans are so overweight that their health is threatened.[40] Hippocrates' dictum that the fat die sooner than the thin rings as true today as it did 2,000 years ago. Indeed, being slightly underweight actually confers some health advantages.

Fortunately, obesity and its ill-effects can usually be totally reversed. Diabetes and hypertension often disappear along with excess weight. Data from life insurance companies show that when obese people lose and keep off weight, their life expectancy rises to what it would have been had they never been obese.

35

Overfeeding early in life can produce extra fat cells that then contribute to obesity for the rest of a person's life. At least four out of five obese children become obese adults. One factor that many nutritionists feel has led to a higher incidence of obesity among children is the substitution of bottle feeding for breast feeding. Mothers who force their babies to finish their bottles may be encouraging more than baby fat.[41]

Some obese children habitually eat too much, but studies have shown that low physical activity often figures centrally in their weight gains as well. Many overweight children do not eat much more than their classmates do, but they are more apt to be inactive, a habit that usually continues later in life.[42] Yet why the obese are so inactive remains a mystery at present.

Crash diets undertaken at any age, however effective in the short term, are unlikely to be beneficial over the long term unless followed by increased routine physical activity and a permanent reduction in caloric intake. For many, a daily caloric excess equivalent to half a slice of bread or half a glass of beer can result in a weight gain of more than 40 pounds within ten years. A reduction in daily exercise by the equivalent of a ten-minute walk can have the same effect.[43]

In the modern age of mechanical convenience and conveyance, many people engage in so little physical activity that simply eating to the point of feeling satisfied means eating excess calories. Studies show that, in the words of Jean Mayer, "decreasing activity below a certain limit will no longer be accompanied by a decrease in appetite."[44] Thus attention must be given to both sides of the diet-exercise equation: *Homo sapiens* need not be *Homo sedentarius*, so long as his diet is commensurate with his level of physical activity.

Salt and Hypertension

Hypertension, or high blood pressure, is one of the most common illnesses in the world today. The prevalence of hypertension in the affluent nations is well recognized, but few people realize that this disease is now emerging in the sprawling urban areas of the world's poorer countries too. Salt intake, genetic factors, stress, and urbanization all seem to be raising the incidence of hypertension in the boroughs of New York as well as in the *favellas* of São Paulo.

High blood pressure goes undetected in many people, but the ailments it promotes, including coronary heart disease, stroke, congestive heart failure, and kidney disease, are all too obvious when they strike. The extensive Framingham heart study showed that two out of every three middle-aged people with a history of stroke or coronary heart disease had above-normal blood pressure.

Hypertension can shorten its victims' lives. A 35-year-old American man with blood pressure 14 percent above normal for his age has lost about nine years of his life expectancy. A 45-year-old man whose blood pressure is 17 percent or more above normal is running twice the risk of a heart attack and four times the risk of a stroke that a man with blood pressure slightly lower than normal faces.[45]

In nearly all cases the actual cause of hypertension is unknown. But dietary factors, especially salt intake levels, are now the subject of many medical studies. Past research has firmly established the link between high salt consumption and high blood pressure in rats. Though the evidence is only circumstantial, it strongly suggests that high salt intake contributes significantly to hypertension in humans as well.

The late Dr. Lewis K. Dahl, who studied hypertension in rats as well as in human beings, found that a low-salt diet drove down blood pressure levels not only for hypertensives in general, but also for obese people in particular. Obesity has been clearly established as a risk factor for both coronary heart disease and hypertension, and obese people who adopt special low-salt diets reduce their blood pressure readings long before they reduce their body weight. Studies of people in the Bahamas, South Africa, Japan, and Polynesia have all shown links between high salt intake and high blood pressure.[46]

The average person in an industrial country consumes at least ten times more salt than the body actually requires.[47] However, some individuals consume large amounts of salt without ever developing hypertension. Dahl and others postulate, and have determined experimentally in rats, that genetic predisposition plays a key role in this process. Thus, some individuals may be so predisposed to hypertension that only a small amount of salt is needed to produce the disease. At the other extreme, those who are not so predisposed may be able to use as much salt as they please without fear of consequences.

The hypertension rates within a country or among different peoples may vary with salt consumption levels. In Japan, where northerners eat more salt than do southerners, the greater incidence of hypertension in the North is apparently salt-related. On the average, Japanese have perhaps the world's highest salt consumption rate, which probably explains their exceptional susceptibility to hypertension and strokes. In New Guinea, a study of the rural highland people showed uniformly low blood pressure levels; but migrants who had moved to the city of Port Moresby suffered from dangerously high blood pressure. Here, rising salt consumption rates are believed to be a contributing factor.[48]

Some doctors believe that a difference in salt consumption rates helps explain why proportionately more U.S. blacks than U.S. whites suffer from hypertension, but dietary surveys to support such a relationship have not been carried out. Twenty-two percent of blacks, compared to 15 percent of the white population, have dangerously elevated blood pressure. Other researchers explain the high incidence of hypertension among blacks as a consequence of life in the urban ghetto and of abnormal stress. Many feel that stress and high salt intake work together insidiously to promote hypertension.[49]

Work-related tedium and stress, as well as some minerals found in drinking water, can apparently produce abnormally high blood pressure.[50] Genetic factors also seem to determine individual susceptibility to hypertension: a child with a hypertensive parent is more apt to develop the disease than a child from a family without hypertension. Also, for unknown reasons, older children in large families tend to have higher blood pressure than their younger sisters and brothers.

Though obvious uncertainties shroud its cause, hypertension can often be controlled easily and painlessly with modern drugs. Yet, by carefully avoiding the risk factors, and by paying special attention to daily salt intake, genetically predisposed people might well completely avoid the disease.

Developing Diabetes

As the affluent diet has spread, the incidence of diabetes has risen throughout the world. In poor countries, diabetes appears to be mainly an urban disease; in rich countries, it afflicts urban and rural residents alike.

In the United States in 1900, diabetes was the twenty-seventh most common cause of death. In the mid-1970s, it has captured fifth place. According to the U.S. National Commission on Diabetes, the number of reported cases in the United States jumped 50 percent in the eight-year period from 1965 to 1973. If the heart diseases, circulatory problems, kidney disorders and other potentially fatal complications of diabetes are added to its annual direct death toll, diabetes emerges as the third most important killer, trailing only cardiovascular disease and cancer. In the United States and the United Kingdom, the disease is also a major cause of blindness.[51]

Puerto Rico, which has undergone rapid economic growth and urbanization, now faces a serious public health threat from diabetes and other degenerative diseases. Even while Puerto Rico's overall health picture improved dramatically, diabetes rose from twelfth to eighth place as a cause of death between 1964 and 1974.

A rich urban resident in India, surveys show, is about twice as likely to develop diabetes as is his poor rural countryman. A similar trend among those people who have only recently been exposed to the affluent lifestyle of the capital city was discovered by a medical researcher in Dakar, Senegal. The number of diabetics in Dakar's clinics increased from 21 to 963 between the years 1965 and 1970.[52]

Many people think of diabetes as a childhood disease that has been brought under control through the use of insulin. In fact, insulin has prolonged the life of juvenile diabetics, but its ready availability has not prevented a tremendous increase in the number of middle-aged or elderly victims of what is called the "maturity-onset" variety of the disease. Juvenile diabetics usually have such low levels of insulin that they could not live without regular injections of this protein. But maturity-onset diabetics often have only slightly deficient levels that are highly influenced by the amount and type of food consumed. Whereas genetic background is of overwhelming importance in the juvenile variety, environmental change and overeating also seem to be associated with maturity-onset diabetes. Yet, the cause of diabetes is not known.

In many countries the incidence of the late-blooming type of diabetes is about four times greater than the incidence of the juvenile type, and the margin is widening. The number of maturity-onset victims in Japan in the last two decades of rapid economic growth has increased noticeably, but cases of juvenile diabetes among Japanese who are 39 or younger are no more frequent than they were twenty years ago. Diabetes was extremely rare among middle-aged Japanese females at the end of World War II, but had become the eighth leading cause of death among this age group by 1972.[53]

Obesity apparently facilitates the emergence of diabetes in those people who are genetically predisposed to the disease. Dietary influences tend to act as catalysts for diabetes in such individuals. Dr. George Cahill, Chief of the Joslin Diabetes Research Center in Boston, recently stressed the catalytic role of overeating, saying: "Overnutrition unmasks the diabetic. The greatest portion of the diabetes we have here in this country is frankly due just to overnutrition." A person who is 20 percent overweight is more than twice as likely to develop diabetes as is a person of normal weight.[54]

Some researchers now suspect that the maturity-onset variety of diabetes can be induced by a sugar-laden diet. Not only does high sugar intake put direct stress on the insulin-producing system of the body, but it can also foster obesity. For those genetically susceptible to diabetes, reducing food consumption, eating less sugar, and losing weight may help prevent this unwanted offspring of the affluent diet.

Diet and Cancer

People who think about a link between diet and cancer often think only about chemical food-additives. Synthetic additives pose real enough problems, but research over the last quarter century is pointing to other, as yet only dimly perceived, dietary factors that may influence cancer rates far more. Under suspicion are dietary aspects that, in some cases, were scarcely even considered by most nutritionists in the past: the degree to which foods are processed, the role of fats in the diet, food storage practices, deficiencies or surpluses of trace elements and vitamins, and even the type of preparation some foods receive.

Worldwide, all dietary factors together outstrip even tobacco as a contributor to cancer. Current evidence, says Dr. Ernst L. Wynder, president of the American Health Foundation, relates diet to "as much as 50 percent of all cancers in women and one-third of all cancers in men."[55] Since about one in every four people in the industrial countries develops cancer, and one in five people dies from it, the toll of diet-related cancers looks large indeed.

Not surprisingly, dietary influences are thought to promote cancers of the digestive system, which includes the mouth, throat, esophagus, stomach, colon, and rectum. Less obviously, diet has also been associated with some cancer sites outside the digestive tract, such as the female breast and the male prostate gland. Both the quantity and quality of food consumed affect the body's hormonal secretions and overall metabolism, in turn affecting a surprising variety of organs.

Though more and more researchers are linking dietary factors with various kinds of cancer, scientists cannot agree upon the exact nature of those links. A case in point is the current debate over the cause of cancers of the bowel (the colon and rectum). Though rare in the rest of the world, bowel cancer is one of the leading killers in the developed Western nations, second only to lung cancer as a source of cancer deaths in the United Kingdom and the United States. The striking international differences in incidence must stem from environmental rather than genetic factors: Japanese who migrate to the United States succumb to bowel cancer at the high U.S. rates, rather than at the low Japanese ones.

"Worldwide, all dietary factors together
outstrip even tobacco as a contributor
to cancer."

Two theories on the causes of bowel cancer, one centered on dietary fiber and the other on dietary fat, have gained wide credence in recent years. Either or both may be correct to some degree; neither has been indisputably established. The subject of popular books and countless magazine and newspaper articles, the fiber theory has recently received widespread publicity. It seems logical; but then, so did many past theories that have long since been discredited. **41**

Fiber, or roughage, has not been defined precisely; but it is usually thought of as the indigestible part of plant cell walls that is present mainly in the outer layers of grain kernels and in raw or lightly cooked fruits and vegetables. Roughage adds bulk to the diet; it also absorbs water and swells in the stomach and intestines. The stools of those with high-fiber diets are softer, larger, and tend to pass through the body more quickly than the harder stools often associated with a low-roughage diet. The consumption-to-elimination process often lasts three or more days for Westerners, whose diet contains less fiber than it once did, while it averages only a day or two for traditional African villagers, whose diet is high in fiber and among whom bowel cancer is rare.

Bowel cancer is caused, many believe, by carcinogenic substances produced by bacteria in the colon. A highly refined diet may alter the composition of the colonic bacteria, encouraging those species that are most likely to degrade digestive substances into carcinogens. Since the low-fiber stool remains in the bowel longer, natural intestinal bacteria have more time to create carcinogens in any case. Finally, the relatively dense low-fiber stool may expose the colon wall to higher concentrations of these carcinogens.[56]

Critics have pointed out several weaknesses in the fiber theory. That the actual concentration of carcinogens in the stool is higher with a refined diet has not been proven to the satisfaction of many. And a faster rate of stool passage through the colon does not necessarily mean that any particular point on the colon wall receives less exposure to carcinogens; the net effect of frequent short exposures could be as great as that of fewer, longer exposures. Most damaging of all to the theory are the results of the few available surveys comparing the diets and cancer rates of various populations.

While bowel cancer does indeed tend to be far more common in countries with affluent diets than in developing countries, a comparison of populations in 37 countries revealed no statistically significant correlation between average fiber intake and colon-cancer rates. Similarly, a study in Hawaii of rising bowel-cancer rates among Japanese immigrants and their children failed to uncover a statistical correlation between dietary fiber and cancer trends.[57] The inadequate definition and measurement of fiber, and the resultant muddled state of international statistics on fiber consumption, may conceal a true connection. But until statistical comparisons reveal a meaningful pattern, a cause-and-effect relationship between fiber and cancer cannot be proven.

The argument that higher fat consumption rather than lower fiber consumption promotes bowel cancer rests upon somewhat firmer empirical foundations, but it, too, can only be called a promising hypothesis at this stage. Some scientists contend that high-fat foods change the composition of intestinal bacteria and promote the production of bile acids that are degraded into carcinogens within the colon.[58] The 37-country comparison just noted revealed that fat and animal protein were more clearly linked to colon-cancer rates than were any other variables measured. The study of Japanese immigrants in Hawaii found a correlation between the consumption of meat and legumes, beef and string beans in particular, and bowel-cancer incidence. The focus on beef, a major source of fats, fits in with fat theories and adds a rider. Beef is higher in saturated fats than other kinds of meat are. Thus the particular type of fat consumed could matter greatly. But how legumes might contribute to bowel cancer, if indeed they do, is not known.

Breast cancer appears internationally in almost exactly the same pattern as bowel cancer. It strikes more women in the United States and Western Europe than any other malignancy, yet is comparatively rare throughout the developing world. While Japanese women seldom develop breast tumors, their chances of doing so begin to rise when they move to the United States and adopt a new way of life.

The close international correlation of bowel and breast-cancer rates is apparently no coincidence. Both rates seem tied to the Western lifestyle, and diet is increasingly suspected as an important contributor to breast-cancer rates, though the evidence is not so clearcut as it is for bowel cancer. Breast-cancer risk correlates with a variety of non-dietary factors: family medical history, income (the wealthier being more susceptible), and the age at which women bear their first child (childless or late-bearing women having the higher risk).

The same study of 37 countries that associated bowel cancer with the high intake of fat and animal protein disclosed that the same kind of diet can be linked to breast cancer. Other studies of human populations (such as vegetarian Seventh-Day Adventists) and of animals have also suggested a relationship between fat intake and breast cancer. The fat content of the diet alters the body's balance of sex hormones, and hormones may in turn affect breast-cancer susceptibility.

Breast cancer is the most common of several kinds of cancer, including those of the prostate gland and testis among men, and those of the ovary, uterus, and uterine lining among women, that are sometimes grouped together under the heading of "endocrine-dependent cancers." These cancers all seem to be influenced by the hormones secreted by the endocrine system, and are quite prevalent in the Western countries. In the United States, breast cancer kills more women than any other cancer does, while prostate cancer follows only lung and bowel cancer as a cause of death among men.

Cancer statistics generally invite only cautious interpretation, and the international pattern in which endocrine-dependent cancers occur is not uniform enough to allow identification of a simple cause. Nevertheless, diet seems to exert an influence on the incidence of these malignancies. Dr. John W. Berg of the University of Iowa concludes:

> The most plausible hypothesis, although based on extremely incomplete knowledge, is that some components of the Western high-protein, high-fat diet acting in early life make individuals prone to develop these cancers. . . . In speculation one could go as far as to suggest that mankind generally evolved under conditions of prudent (i.e., low-fat and protein) nutrition and that the present affluent diet from childhood onward may overstimulate the endocrine system, producing the same effect that one would obtain running a diesel engine on high-octane airplane fuel.

While obesity is associated with cancers of the uterine lining and kidney in females, the most widespread influences of overnutrition on cancer seem to stem from the richness, not the quantity, of food that typifies the affluent diet.[59]

Though the general incidence of cancer has risen ominously over the last half century, that of stomach cancer has declined markedly in the United States and in several European countries. Recently, stomach cancer has also begun to decline in some countries still having exceptionally high rates, including Japan, where the incidence is the world's highest. This global decline has been one of the most pronounced cancer trends of this century, yet its cause eludes cancer researchers. Most scientists look to diet for the underlying explanation, but the exact combination of factors causing the drop is simply not known. In a world fraught with many pernicious cancer mysteries, these benevolent unknown forces offer some solace.

Particular foods and cultural practices seem to invite stomach cancer. Moreover, one's birthplace may help determine one's cause of death. First-generation international migrants get stomach cancer at the same rate as their native countrymen. Such findings call attention to the paramount importance of environmental exposures early in life, but no single factor has been identified as common to all regions in which stomach cancer is prevalent.

Several different factors have been isolated as possible contributors to the exceptional incidence of stomach cancer in Japan. A national penchant for dried, salted fish and pickled vegetables is one; many believe that the nitrosamines, known carcinogens that are often found in these foods, are the main culprits. Asbestos residues on talc-coated white rice, without which no Japanese meal is complete, could also be cancer-promoting. The mountains of smoked fish consumed each year in Japan, which usually contain chemicals called polycyclic aromatic hydrocarbons that have long been known to be carcinogenic in other contexts, may be a cancer agent. Internationally, all populations consuming large amounts of smoked fish have high rates of stomach cancer.[60]

Much recent speculation has centered on nitrosamines as the main agents responsible for stomach cancer.[61] However, direct consumption of these dangerous chemicals poses a less formidable problem than the chemical combinations in food and water, the methods of food treatment, and the overall dietary patterns that allow the body to manufacture them. Nitrite, which can combine with other food components to form nitrosamines, occurs naturally in saliva. But salivary nitrite concentration may be influenced by the level of nitrite or nitrate ingested. The water supplies in parts of England, Japan, Israel, Chile, and Colombia where stomach-cancer incidence is high have been found to contain strong concentrations of nitrates; high natural nitrate levels in the soils of these regions may also mean that locally-produced food is nitrate-rich. The use of fertilizers containing nitrates can also boost the nitrate content of food. Finally, small amounts of nitrates and nitrites are often added to fish and cured-meat products as preservatives.

Nitrate is not dangerous unless it converts to nitrite. Since food refrigeration is known to inhibit this conversion, the gradual spread of electrical home-refrigeration in this century could conceivably be driving down stomach-cancer rates. So could the year-round availability of vitamin-rich fresh fruits, lettuce, and other fresh leafy vegetables; the vitamin C they contain, which inhibits the formation of nitrosamines, has been associated with lower odds of developing stomach cancer.

The geographic and cultural patchwork of esophageal-cancer zones is even more perplexing than the erratic stomach-cancer pattern. The incidence of esophageal cancer varies wildly among countries, within countries, and by sex within specific regions. Unfortunately, though, malignancies of the esophagus have become more frequent in several countries over the last few decades.

Especially bewildering to scientists is the distribution of esophageal cancer in Central Asia, where—Persian writings from 1100 A.D. inform us—this affliction is no newcomer. Exceptionally high rates occur near the Caspian coast of Iran, but among groups living within a 300-mile stretch the incidence varies as much as thirtyfold for women and sixfold for men. The zone of high risk encompasses Iran, northern China, and the Soviet republics of Turkmenia, Kazakhstan, and Uzbekistan. An office of the U.N.'s International Agency for

Research on Cancer has been established in Iran to seek the causes of this curious cancer mosaic.[62]

In Africa, esophageal cancer also appears in unusual geographic patterns. While the disease is rare in West Africa, several areas of southern and eastern Africa have experienced a dramatic rise in esophageal cancer over the last 40 years—a rise comparable to the rise of lung cancer in the industrial countries. The most promising explanation put forward so far associates the increased incidence of this cancer with the increased consumption of maize-based beer in this century. Some unidentified product of the fermentation process may be carcinogenic.[63]

Associations between alcohol consumption and esophageal cancer have been established in the United States, France, Puerto Rico, and Northern Europe.[64] Alcohol consumption alone boosts the risk, as does cigarette smoking alone, but the really big jump in susceptibility comes when heavy drinking and smoking are combined. In the United States, moderate smokers who drink heavily are 25 times more likely to develop esophageal cancer than are those who do not drink. Though overall U.S. rates for this cancer are low, black Americans, particularly northern urban blacks, have suffered a sharp, unexplained rise in the incidence of esophageal cancer since 1940.

Alcohol consumption affects the mouth and throat as well as the esophagus. Heavy drinkers in the United States are from two to six times more likely than non-drinkers to contract mouth and throat cancers, with the precise risk dependent on smoking habits. Alcohol and tobacco consumption together are responsible for three-fourths of all oral cavity cancers in U.S. males. Alcoholics are subject to cancer of the larynx, or voice box, far more frequently than are non-alcoholics—again, smoking multiplies the risk. They also are more prone to contract liver cancer, which often follows upon the heels of cirrhosis, an inflammatory disease of the liver that mainly afflicts heavy drinkers.

Though the varied ingredients or impurities in different liquors apparently have effects on one potential cancer site or another, the balance of evidence strongly indicates that heavy alcohol consumption per se boosts cancer risks. Both human disease patterns and the

"Two-thirds of all cancers associated
with combinations of alcohol and tobacco
could be prevented by eliminating
smoking."

results of experiments on animals suggest that alcohol is not directly
carcinogenic, but rather enhances the carcinogenic impact of other
agents. One striking conclusion is that two-thirds of all cancers associated with combinations of alcohol and tobacco consumption
could be prevented by eliminating smoking.[65]

47

Quite by chance, following the mysterious deaths of 100,000 turkeys
in the United Kingdom in 1960, a powerful natural carcinogen that
often finds its way into human food was discovered. Aflatoxin, the
product of a certain mold that can grow on peanuts, grains, and other
foods, has achieved a dubious distinction as one of the most potent
known carcinogens in rats. It has been implicated in human cancers,
especially liver cancer, as well.

The mold that produces aflatoxin thrives under sustained moist
warmth, and is therefore most common in tropical countries. The
discovery of aflatoxin's deadly power and the subsequent analysis
of market foods for aflatoxin content over the last decade may in
turn finally explain the previously unfathomable high incidence of
liver cancer in patchy areas throughout the tropics. Aflatoxin con-
tamination has been correlated with liver cancer rates in parts of Ken-
ya, Mozambique (where the world's highest incidence of liver cancer
is found), Swaziland, the Ivory Coast, Thailand, and the Philippines.[66] Aflatoxin can, under the right conditions, accumulate in
foods in temperate zones as well as in the tropics. Since its presence
in internationally traded products is always possible, food inspectors
everywhere are being forced to redouble their vigilance.

No review of dietary influences on cancer would be complete without
mention of synthetic food-additives and residues. Though human-
made chemicals in food constitute only a small part of the diet-cancer
complex, their exact contribution to cancer rates is a conspicuous unknown, and some unpleasant surprises are probably in store. The only certainty is that citizens in the more economically developed countries ingest a few thousand different chemical compounds, a majority
of which have not yet been adequately tested for links to cancer, genetic mutations, birth defects, or behavioral problems.

Suspect food additives are being scrutinized in laboratories and a
few additives once assumed safe have been removed from use in one

country or another. But, unfortunately, the global testing capacity remains overtaxed by the need to evaluate suspicious new and old substances of all kinds. Newly introduced additives are subjected to fairly rigorous testing, but once a product has taken its place in the food industry and in cultural life, its removal becomes far more difficult politically. When test results are ambiguous, as they often are, and the probability of cancerous effects on human beings appears slight, as it often does, the economic and political pressure to give a profitable product the benefit of the doubt can seem irresistible.

In addition to the obvious need to detect and remove carcinogenic contaminants from food, what implications for public policy emerge from this review of dietary influences on cancer? The principal policy prescription, however lackluster, must be the continuation and the expansion of research designed to identify meaningful associations between specific dietary traits and specific cancers. Ideally, risky habits will be clearly identified even before the biological mechanisms of cancer are understood, permitting those so choosing to cut their odds of developing cancer. Many such research efforts will have to be oriented towards specific locales, since a wide range of local circumstances appears to surround diet-related cancers. No conspicuous villain—no dietary equivalent of the cigarette—is in sight; no simple explanation for the morass of evidence on diet and the multitude of malignancies it influences has presented itself.

Some U.S. cancer researchers wonder whether their identification of the cancer risks associated with the high-fat, refined Western diet is certain enough to warrant publicizing the potential benefits of dietary changes. A growing number, however, now recommend the adoption of a "prudent diet" to help reduce cancer risk, much as heart specialists have long recommended dietary changes for potential heart attack victims without absolute proof of the benefits.[67] The strength of the case for any given food's influence on cancer remains weaker than the cardiologists' dietary case. But the argument for trying to prevent cancer through dietary changes gains appeal in view of the happy coincidence in dietary directions called for by current knowledge of both heart disease and cancer. Reduced consumption of fats, especially animal fats, and increased consumption of whole grains, fresh fruits, and vegetables, appear to be just what the doctor should order.

National Nutrition Strategies

Throughout history, food-consumption patterns have been influenced by many forces, but health considerations have not always been among them. Long lacking both the medical knowledge and the agricultural resources needed to promote healthy diets, humanity now has both, and the marked reduction of malnutrition of any type is within the reach of governments seriously committed to that end. Nutrition strategies, with which governments try to give a coherent and positive shape to the forces molding people's diets, are increasingly recognized as a public responsibility. In a growing number of poor countries, the idea of national planning for improved nutrition has already caught on, though much remains to be done. In the industrial countries, health officials and some politicians are voicing the need for dietary health strategies, but only Norway and Sweden have moved toward systematic health-oriented nutrition policies.

Observing the strong correlation between poverty and undernutrition, some analysts see nutrition strategies as an unnecessary diversion from the overriding task of raising the incomes of the poor. According to various versions of this view, hastening economic growth, redistributing income, or both are the best defenses against undernutrition. While such arguments stand on obvious truths, they can be dangerously misleading. Creating minimum income levels is certainly a necessary part of a strategy for stamping out undernutrition, but it is seldom sufficient in itself to complete the task. While the poor must have land, jobs, and decent incomes if undernutrition is to be wiped out, the positive impact of all three on diets can be enhanced when combined with a good nutrition plan.

At the rate of economic growth realistically foreseeable in many poor countries, decades or even centuries will pass before undernutrition ceases to be a serious threat. Moreover, if the economic growth patterns now prevailing in many countries persist, the landless, the small-scale farmers, and the urban slum-dwellers, among others, may derive little benefit from increases in the gross national product—even when these increases take the form of agricultural production. The GNP is simply not an adequate gauge of progress in meeting human needs.

For example, Brazilian farmers have taken advantage of the tight world protein market by rapidly increasing their production of soybeans, most of which are sold abroad as livestock feed. But to achieve the lucrative boom, farmers planted soybeans on land that had been used to grow the traditional bean crop—the staple protein food eaten by low-income families. Per capita production of this food bean in Brazil fell by one-third between 1971 and 1974, and the price tripled. In effect, rich European and Japanese consumers bid protein away from the poor of Brazil. The Brazilian GNP received a healthy boost, national foreign-exchange reserves were bolstered, and soybean farmers prospered—but undernutrition doubtlessly grew more severe among the Brazilian poor.

One way countries can help assure that nutritional considerations receive high priority is to establish a government agency that both monitors the nutrition of the population and weighs the nutritional implications of major policies and programs. Analyses of the nutritional impacts of various institutions and projects could conceivably help poor countries avoid or alter development paths, such as Brazil's recent soybean boom, that would likely entail negative health repercussions. At the least, those in power would be forced to confront openly the human consequences of the programs they pursue. On the more positive side, systematic nutritional scanning can help keep a spotlight on programs needed to improve diets—whether land reforms, food supplements, or the provision of jobs. Documentation of hardship and inequity can itself right no wrongs, but it is a critical first step. In the United States, for example, the shocking findings of nutritional surveys in the late 1960s prompted the government to expand substantially its food-assistance programs for the poor.

Nutrition planning is not a surrogate for economic growth, but setting nutritional priorities can help give growth a human face. Nor is a nutrition strategy a substitute for fundamental reforms in the distribution of land and income. Such a strategy can, however, perhaps spur a redistribution of productive resources. Where growing populations are overwhelming the local environment and food-production capacity, nutrition planning cannot substitute for a cut in the birth rate. But it can prompt policymakers to accord higher priority to the family planning services, education, medical care, and improved diets that promote reduced family size.

Besides these influences that nutrition planning can conceivably have on the broad shape of national development, specific nutritional programs that have already proven effective in various poor countries deserve consideration in others. Just as fortifying bread, milk, and salt wiped out many vitamin-deficiency diseases in the West, adding nutrients to various foods is paying off in many poor countries today. For example, iodized salt has greatly reduced goiter in Guatemala, and protein-fortified bread is combatting malnutrition in urban areas of India and the Philippines. Yet the potential for fortification is far from fully realized. Special efforts to provide food supplements to needy infants and to pregnant and nursing mothers may be the most critical need of all, given the evidence that lasting damage to learning ability and health can result from undernutrition early in life.

Nutrition education—for doctors and other adults as well as for children—usually has a dramatic payoff among people at any income level. The World Health Organization estimates that one-half or more of the nutritional problems of Africa could be solved through appropriate education. There and elsewhere, ignorance about the nutritional value of local foods, misconceptions about the appropriateness of certain diets for infants and pregnant women, and traditional food-allocation patterns within the family are all causes of undernutrition.[68] A campaign to halt the disastrous decline in breast feeding by educating doctors and mothers, controlling irresponsible advertising of commercially prepared infant foods, and providing nurseries in women's workplaces is also critically needed in many countries of Africa, Asia, and Latin America. Finally, the better-off in poor countries should be made aware of the dangers of the affluent diet before they repeat all the mistakes made by people in Europe and North America.

In more affluent countries, fortification programs, generally high incomes, and food or income supplements have eliminated most—though by no means all—serious undernutrition. Guaranteed minimum incomes for all the residents in these countries could virtually eradicate undernutrition, and thus could provide a solid foundation

51

for comprehensive nutritional planning designed to combat both under- and overnutrition.

Against the menace of overconsumption, most developed countries have not yet begun to fight. Both medical communities and governments share responsibility for this failure. The overwhelming bulk of medical attention is devoted to the expert treatment of "crises" such as heart attacks, even though these seemingly sudden attacks are often the culmination of decades of nutritional abuse.

Governments, through their agricultural, economic, and educational policies, have at best usually ignored the problems of overnutrition. At worst they have actively promoted unhealthy consumption trends. Most nutrition education efforts dwell on the dwindling deficiency problems of the past rather than on the massive newer dangers of overnutrition, and key agricultural and economic decisions are made with scant regard for their impacts on health. Thus, faced with mountains of surplus butter, the European Economic Community Commission recently proposed taxing edible oils to make margarine as expensive as butter—in effect, to encourage higher consumption of saturated fats. In Great Britain, a recent Government White Paper on national food-production policy ignored health considerations while calling for increased output of milk, beef, and sugar beets.[69] The Congressionally-mandated involvement of the U.S. Department of Agriculture in promoting higher consumption of eggs by Americans provides another such example.

By subsidizing the further growth of food industries whose product, when consumed at current levels, is unhealthy, governments sanction the growth of huge industries with vested interests in promoting bad health. Here, a parallel to the detrimental—and, in many countries, government-subsidized—operations of the tobacco industry might be drawn.

The following changes for those on the affluent diet are recommended by most doctors and nutritionists studying overnutrition and its consequences:

1. Fat consumption should be reduced and held to under 35 percent of total calorie intake, in contrast to the 40-50 percent now common. Moderation in the consumption of meat, dairy products, and fried foods; a shift from beef and pork to poultry and fish; and a preference for grass-fed rather than grain-fed beef can help meet this goal.

2. Whenever possible, saturated fats should be replaced by unsaturated fats. In practice, this means substituting vegetable fats (such as margarine) for animal fats (such as butter).

3. Men especially should radically reduce their cholesterol intake by eating few eggs and only moderate amounts of other livestock products.

4. Sugar and salt intake should be sharply reduced.

5. Consumption of whole grains, potatoes and other starchy foods, and fresh fruits and vegetables should be increased.

6. Personal energy intake and energy expenditure need to be kept in balance, in part by calorie budgeting, and in part by engaging in more physical activity.

Changes like these do not come easily; for many they violate life-long habits and strongly ingrained notions about which foods are healthful and about which ones are tasty. And building exercise into a sedentary lifestyle is difficult for most individuals. Moreover, when people revise their consumption patterns, changes will ripple through the farm and food industries as well—changes unwelcome to those whose businesses are threatened.

A national strategy to counter overnutrition, like one to eliminate undernutrition, must involve a wide range of policies, not all of them directly linked to food and agriculture. In rich as in poor countries, the marketplace has its own set of priorities, and health is not one of them. The object must be to build a structure of economic incentives and institutions that encourages healthy food-production and consumption patterns.

Agricultural research, crop subsidies, taxes, meat-grading, international trade, and medical and general education are among the many concerns that a strategy against overnutrition must encompass. Since overnutrition and lack of exercise are part of the same problem, such topics as recreation and transportation policy enter into the picture as well. The construction of bicycle paths rather than parking lots for urban commuters would create, among other benefits, the opportunity for regular exercise and thereby perhaps reduce the incidence of obesity and heart disease.

Among the industrial countries, Sweden and Norway stand alone in their recent decisions to try to integrate modern dietary health concerns into national economic and agricultural planning. Particularly through a vigorous public education program, the Swedish Government has worked to reduce the amount of calories, fats, sugar, and alcohol Swedes consume and to increase the amount of exercise Swedes get. The Norwegian Government has proposed to its legislature a nutrition and food policy through which it hopes both to increase national self-sufficiency in food supplies and to cut the mounting national toll of cardiovascular and other diet-related diseases.[70]

The Norwegian Government hopes to establish a broad array of subsidies, grants, price policies, and other incentives that will promote a stabilization of meat consumption (which has been rising over the last decade); an increase in fish consumption; a reduction in feed-grain imports; a preference for low-fat over whole milk; and a reversal of the decline in consumption of grains, potatoes, and vegetables. The educational potential of government agencies, private organizations, and schools will be enlisted to inform Norwegians about the health implications of their eating habits. Representatives of the eight different ministries, ranging from Fisheries to Agriculture to Foreign Affairs, whose activities should be influenced by the national nutrition and food plan will meet in a coordinating body. If the plan is implemented, Norway may not only better the health of its populace, but also reduce its agricultural trade deficit and reduce its claims on world food resources.

"The dietary changes called for by the
leading theories of cancer causation are
precisely those that help to reduce the
threats of heart disease and obesity."

Some people, especially representatives of threatened food industries, argue that strategies to alter the affluent diet cannot be justified on scientific grounds. A comprehensive review of dietary impacts on health, however, reveals a persuasive case for dietary change. The geography of the affluent diet and of the diseases it apparently promotes, together with the available experimental evidence, creates a powerful body of circumstantial evidence against this diet.

With afflictions such as coronary heart disease, whose development spans decades and is obviously influenced by many forces, the exact causative role of any one factor necessarily remains elusive. Nevertheless, that aspects of the affluent diet promote atherosclerosis and heart disease, the leading killers in the West, has been proven beyond reasonable doubt. For other diseases, such as cancers of the bowel, breast, and prostate, our understanding of dietary influences is much less advanced. Yet the dietary changes called for by the leading theories of cancer causation are precisely those that help to reduce the threats of heart disease and obesity. It should not be surprising that the same dietary factors—those setting the modern Western diet apart from all others in human history—have been implicated in the origins of many different diseases.

Certainly more remains to be learned about diet and health, but, as Dr. D. M. Hegsted of Harvard University observes of problems of data and proof in this field, "one does not need to know all of the answers before one can make practical recommendations." The dietary changes that doctors are prescribing involve no foreseeable risks to the health of the population; quite the contrary, all evidence points to the great risks involved in clinging to our current diet. The only known risk associated with more prudent diets is to the food industries that would be affected. But, "while these industries deserve some consideration," observes Dr. Hegsted, "their interests cannot supersede the health interest of the population they must feed."[71]

Though the health connection is sufficient by itself to justify programs to alter the diets of the affluent, two other considerations make such changes even more attractive. One is economy in personal food budgets. Reducing meat consumption and substituting vegetable for animal protein sources both save money. Grains, fresh fruits, and vegetables usually cost far less than processed, pre-prepared foods and snacks that tend to be overly refined and loaded with sugar, fats, and unnecessary additives.

56 Second, reducing overnutrition might contribute in a small way to reducing undernutrition. Widespread moderation in the consumption of fatty grain-fed livestock products—the production of which uses up over a third of the world's grain each year—can modify the terms of the global competition between rich and poor for available food and agricultural resources. The competition for agricultural products is sometimes overt, as in the recent case of Brazilian soybeans, but it is usually manifested more subtly in the competition for products in the world marketplace and, ultimately, in the allocation of land and capital.

Few potential social policies promise so many benefits and so few costs as the decision to alter the affluent diet. In the end, only individuals—who must change their behavior—can reduce overnutrition's toll. But governments have a responsibility to provide a structure of incentives and information that enhances rather than threatens the well-being of their populations. In the nineteenth century, as scientists became aware of the role of filth in propagating infectious disease, governments tried to provide clean water and sewage facilities. More recently, the responsibility of governments to combat undernutrition has been widely recognized. Today, our growing knowledge of the health consequences of overnutrition demands another step in the evolution of public health policies.

Notes

1. The latest recommended nutritional requirements are in *Energy and Protein Requirements: Report of a Joint FAO/WHO Ad Hoc Expert Committee* (Rome: Food and Agriculture Organization and World Health Organization, 1973). Nevin S. Scrimshaw, "An Analysis of Past and Present Recommended Dietary Allowances for Protein in Health and Disease," *New England Journal of Medicine*, January 15 and January 27, 1976; and C. Garza, *et al*, "Human Protein Requirements: The Effect of Variations of Energy Intake Within the Maintenance Range," *American Journal of Clinical Nutrition*, March 1976, both suggest the inadequacy of current protein standards.

2. Thomas T. Poleman, "World Food: A Perspective," *Science*, May 9, 1975, critically reviews past global nutrition surveys. Also see United Nations, *Assessment of the World Food Situation, Present and Future* (Rome: U.N. World Food Conference, November 1974).

3. Derrick B. Jelliffe, "Tropical Problems in Nutrition," *Annals of Internal Medicine*, Vol. 79, 1973, p. 701.

4. Jelliffe, "Tropical Problems in Nutrition"; Moisés Béhar, "Poverty Must Take the Blame," *People* (London), Vol. 3, No. 1, 1976. By the commonly used Gomez system of classification, the mildly undernourished weigh 75-90 percent, the moderately undernourished weigh 60-75 percent, and the severely undernourished weigh less than 60 percent of their expected weights according to age.

5. J. J. Bengoa, "The State of World Nutrition," World Health Organization, Geneva, 1973; W. R. Aykroyd, *Conquest of Deficiency Diseases* (Geneva: World Health Organization, 1970); Alfred Sommer, "Xeropthalmia: A Status Report," *Tropical Doctor*, April 1976.

6. Thomas Stapleton, "Child Health in China," *Journal of Tropical Pediatrics and Environmental Child Health*, September 1973; Jay M. Arena, "Nutritional Status of China's Children: An Overview," *Nutrition Reviews*, October 1974.

7. K. V. Bailey, "Malnutrition in the African Region," *WHO Chronicle*, Vol. 29, 1975, p. 354; "Tackling Nutrition Problems in Africa," *WHO Chronicle*, Vol. 30, 1976, p. 28.

8. Pan American Health Organization, "Food and Nutrition Situation in the Latin American and Caribbean Countries," in *Final Report of the 23rd Meeting of the Directing Council of PAHO* (Washington, D. C.: October 1975); Jelliffe, "Tropical Problems in Nutrition."

9. Freeman H. Quimby, "Hunger and Malnutrition in the United States: How Much?" Congressional Research Service, Library of Congress, Washington, D.C., May 1, 1975; Department of Health, Education and Welfare, *Preliminary Findings of the First Health and Nutrition Examination Survey, U. S., 1971-72: Dietary Intake and Biochemical Findings* (Washington, D.C.: G.P.O., January 1974) and *Anthropometric and Clinical Findings* (Washington, D.C.: G.P.O., April 1975).

10. Ruth Rice Puffer and Carlos V. Serrano, *Patterns of Mortality in Childhood* (Washington, D. C.: Pan American Health Organization, 1973).

11. *Ibid.*

12. David Morley, *Paediatric Priorities in the Developing World* (London: Butterworths, 1973); Herbert G. Birch, "Malnutrition, Learning, and Intelligence," *American Journal of Public Health*, Vol. 62, No. 6, 1972.

13. Puffer and Serrano, *Patterns of Mortality in Childhood*; Gerald T. Keusch, "Malnutrition and Infection: Deadly Allies," *Natural History*, November 1975.

14. Keusch, "Malnutrition and Infection."

15. Michael C. Latham, "Nutrition and Infection in National Development," *Science*, May 9, 1975; Morley, *Paediatric Priorities*.

16. Nevin S. Scrimshaw and Moisés Béhar, "Protein Malnutrition in Young Children," *Science*, June 30, 1961.

17. Nevin S. Scrimshaw, Carl E. Taylor, and John E. Gordon, *Interactions of Nutrition and Infection* (Geneva: World Health Organization, 1968).

18. Derrick B. Jelliffe and E. F. Patrice Jelliffe, "Human Milk, Nutrition, and the World Resource Crisis," *Science*, May 9, 1975; Alan Berg, *The Nutrition Factor* (Washington, D. C.: Brookings Institution, 1973).

19. Scrimshaw, Taylor, and Gordon, *Interactions of Nutrition and Infection.*

20. National Academy of Sciences, "The Relationship of Nutrition to Brain Development and Behavior," Washington, D. C., June 1973.

21. Joaquín Cravioto and Elsa DeLicardie, "Environmental Correlates of Severe Clinical Malnutrition and Language Development in Survivors from Kwashiorkor or Marasmus," in *Nutrition, the Nervous System, and Behavior* (Washington, D. C.: Pan American Health Organization, 1972); "Mental Retardation from Malnutrition: 'Irreversible'," *Journal of the American Medical Association*, September 30, 1968.

22. Pek Hien Liang, *et al*, "Evaluation of Mental Development in Relation to Early Malnutrition," *American Journal of Clinical Nutrition*, December 1967. In "Malnutrition, Learning, and Intelligence," Birch reviews numerous studies of undernutrition and intelligence.

23. Roger Lewin, "The Poverty of Undernourished Brains," *New Scientist*, October 24, 1974; John Dobbing, "Lasting Deficits and Distortions of the Adult Brain Following Infantile Undernutrition," in *Nutrition, the Nervous System, and Behavior*.

24. Myron Winick, *et al*, "Malnutrition and Environmental Enrichment by Early Adoption," *Science*, December 19, 1975.

25. National Academy of Sciences, "The Relationship of Nutrition to Brain Development and Behavior"; Roger Lewin, "Starved Brains," *Psychology Today*, September 1975. "Malnutrition and Mental Development," *WHO Chronicle*, Vol. 28, 1974, p. 101, stresses the lack of strong proof that mild undernutrition impairs mental development.

26. Michael C. Latham and Francisco Cobos, "The Effects of Malnutrition on Intellectual Development and Learning," *American Journal of Public Health*, July 1971; Berg, *The Nutrition Factor*.

27. Lars Werko, "Can We Prevent Heart Disease?" *Annals of Internal Medicine*, February 1971; Department of Health, Education, and Welfare, *Monthly Vital Statistics Report*, May 1975; "Special Communication," *Journal of the American Medical Association*, March 4, 1974.

28. S. G. Sarvotham and J. N. Berry, "Prevalence of Coronary Heart Disease in an Urban Population in Northern India," *Circulation*, June 1968; "Heart Disease Problems in China," *Annals of Internal Medicine*, January 1974; World Health Organization, *Second Regional Seminar on Cardiovascular Diseases* (Manila: 1975).

29. World Health Organization, "Report on the Epidemiology, Control and Management of Coronary Heart Disease in Nepal," New Delhi, June 19, 1974; E. Bertrand, *et al*, "La Maladie Coronaire en Côte d'Ivoire," *Semaine des Hôpitaux de Paris*, Vol. 50, 1974, p. 1871; "Sû Corazon es su Salud," *Boletin de la Oficina Sanitaria Panamericana*, April 1972.

30. *World Health Statistics Annual, 1972*, Vol. 1 (Geneva: World Health Organization, 1975).

31. W. B. Kannel, *et al*, "Factors of Risk in the Development of Coronary Heart Disease: Six Year Follow-up Experience, The Framingham Study," *Annals of Internal Medicine*, Vol. 55, No. 33, 1961; American Heart Association, "Heart Facts," New York, 1973.

32. E. Personen, *et al*, "Thickenings in the Coronary Arteries in Infancy as an Indication of Genetic Factors in Coronary Heart Disease," *Circulation*, February 1975.

33. Kannel, "Factors of Risk"; Committee on Nutrition, "Childhood Diet and Coronary Heart Disease," *Pediatrics*, February 1972.

34. Food and Nutrition Board of the National Academy of Sciences and Council on Food and Nutrition of the American Medical Association, "Diet and Coronary Heart Disease," Washington, D.C., July 1972.

35. H. I. Russek, "Behaviour Patterns, Stress, and Coronary Heart Disease," *American Family Physician*, April 1974.

36. National Board of Health and Welfare, *Diet and Health* (Stockholm: 1972); R. A. Shorey, *et al*, "Efficacy of Diet and Exercise in the Reduction of Serum Cholesterol and Triglycerides in Free-Living Adult Males," *American Journal of Clinical Nutrition*, May 1976; Advisory Panel of the Committee on Medical Aspects of Food Policy on Diet in Relation to Cardiovascular and Cerebrovascular Disease, *Diet and Coronary Heart Disease* (London: Her Majesty's Stationary Office, 1974).

37. American Heart Association, "Diet and Coronary Heart Disease," New York, 1973; R. M. Feeley, *et al*, "Cholesterol Content of Foods," *Journal of the American Dietetic Association*, Vol. 61, 1972, p. 134.

38. Jean Mayer, "The Bitter Truth About Sugar," *New York Times Magazine*, June 20, 1976.

39. M. E. Moore, *et al*, "Obesity, Social Class and Mental Illness," *Journal of the American Medical Association*, Vol. 181, 1962, p. 138; Jean Mayer, ed., *U. S. Nutrition Policies in the Seventies* (San Francisco: Freeman and Co., 1973).

40. R. S. Goodhart, ed., *Modern Nutrition in Health and Disease* (Philadelphia: Lea and Febiger, 1973); "Overweight: Its Prevention and Significance," reprints from *Statistical Bulletin*, Metropolitan Life Insurance Company, New York, 1960; "Statement of Dr. Theodore Cooper," in U.S. Senate, Select Committee on Nutrition and Human Needs, *Diet Related to Killer Diseases*, Hearings, July 27-28, 1976.

41. R. K. Oates, "Infant Feeding Practices," *British Medical Journal*, 1973 (Vol. 2), p. 762.

42. Jean Mayer, "Hidden Bonds: Obesity, Heredity, and Hunger," *World Health*, February 1974.

43. Eunice Tsomondo and Jim Jones, "Obesity: A Disease of Indolence and Affluence," *Central African Journal of Medicine*, January 1974.

44. Mayer, "Hidden Bonds."

45. Ray Gifford, Jr., "Hypertension 1975," *Drug Therapy*, May 1975; American Heart Association, "Heart Facts."

46. Lewis K. Dahl, "Salt and Hypertension," *American Journal of Clinical Nutrition*, February 1972; L. C. Isaacson, "Sodium Intake and Hypertension," *Lancet*, 1963 (Vol. 1), p. 946.

47. R. L. Weinsier, "Overview: Salt and the Development of Essential Hypertension," *Preventive Medicine*, March 1976.

48. Naosuke Sasaki, "High Blood Pressure and the Salt Intake of the Japanese," *Japanese Heart Journal*, July 1962; A. G. Shaper, "Cardiovascular Disease in the Tropics," *British Medical Journal*, September 30, 1972.

49. E. Harburg, *et al*, "Socio-Ecological Stress, Suppressed Hostility, Skin Color, and Black-White Male Blood Pressure: Detroit," *Psychosomatic Medicine*, July-August 1973; Joseph Eyer, "Hypertension as a Disease of Modern Society," *International Journal of Health Services*, Vol. 5, No. 4, 1975.

50. W. E. Morton, "Hypertension and Drinking Water Constituents in Colorado," *American Journal of Public Health*, July 1971.

51. U. S. Senate, Select Committee on Nutrition and Human Needs, *Nutrition and Diseases—1974*, Part 4, Hearings, February 26, 1974; *Report of the National Commission on Diabetes to the Congress of the United States*, Vol. 1 (Washington, D. C.: National Institutes of Health, 1975).

61

62

52. *Yearly Report of Vital Statistics—1974*, (San Juan, Puerto Rico: Division of Vital Statistics, 1974); R. V. Sattre, "The Problem of Diabetes Mellitus in India," *Journal of the Indian Medical Association*, July 1, 1973; M. Sankalé, "Les Particularites du Diabetes Sucré chez le Noir Africain," *Journées de Diabetologie de l'Hôtel Dieu*, May 1971.

53. N. Kuzuye and K. Kosaka, "Diabetics in Japan," in *Symposium on Diabetes in Asian People*, Proceedings of the 13th Annual Meeting of the Japanese Diabetic Society, Kumomoto, May 22, 1970.

54. D. Rimoin, "Inheritance in Diabetes Mellitus," *Medical Clinics of North America*, July 1971; U. S. Senate, *Nutrition and Diseases—1974;* "Statement of Dr. Theodore Cooper."

55. Ernst L. Wynder, "Introductory Remarks," *Cancer Research*, November 1975.

56. Denis P. Burkitt, "Some Neglected Leads to Cancer Causation," *Journal of the National Cancer Institute*, November 1971; D. P. Burkitt, A. R. P. Walker, and N.S. Painter, "Effect of Dietary Fibre on Stools and Transit-Time, and Its Role in the Causation of Disease," *Lancet*, December 30, 1972.

57. G. S. Drasar and Doreen Irving, "Environmental Factors and Cancer of the Colon and Breast," *British Journal of Cancer*, Vol. 27, 1973, p. 167; William Haenszel, *et al*, "Large-Bowel Cancer in Hawaiian Japanese," *Journal of the National Cancer Institute*, December 1973.

58. M. J. Hill, "Colon Cancer: A Disease of Fibre Depletion or of Dietary Excess," *Digestion*, 1974 (Vol. 2), p. 289; Ernst L. Wynder, "The Epidemiology of Large Bowel Cancer," *Cancer Research*, November 1975.

59. John W. Berg, "Can Nutrition Explain the Pattern of International Epidemiology of Hormone-Dependent Cancers?" *Cancer Research*, November 1975; Ernst L. Wynder, "On the Key Importance of Nutrition in Cancer Causation and Prevention," presented to the American Cancer Society's Sixteenth Science Writers Seminar, St. Augustine, Florida, March 22-27, 1974.

60. John W. Berg, "Diet," in Joseph F. Fraumeni, Jr., ed., *Persons at High Risk of Cancer* (New York: Academic Press, 1976).

61. Pelayo Correa, *et al*, "A Model for Gastric Cancer Epidemiology," *Lancet*, July 12, 1975; John H. Weisburger and Ronald Raineri, "Dietary Factors and the Etiology of Gastric Cancer," *Cancer Research*, November 1975; Robert Zaldivar and Harry Robinson, "Epidemiological Investigation on Stomach Cancer Mortality in Chileans: Association with Nitrate Fertilizer," *Zeitschrift für Krebsforschung*, Vol. 80, 1973, p. 289; M. J. Hill, G. Hawksworth, and G. Tattersall, "Bacteria, Nitrosamines and Cancer of the Stomach," *British Journal of Cancer*, Vol. 28, 1973, p. 562.

62. H. Hormozdiari, *et al*, "Dietary Factors and Esophageal Cancer in the Caspian Littoral of Iran," *Cancer Research*, November 1975.

63. Paula Cook, "Cancer of the Esophagus in Africa," *British Journal of Cancer*, Vol. 25, 1971, p. 853; "Oesophageal Carcinoma in Africa," *Lancet*, March 18, 1972.

64. Kenneth J. Rothman, "Alcohol," in Fraumeni, *Persons at High Risk; International Agency for Research on Cancer, Annual Report 1975* (Lyon, France: 1975).

65. Rothman, "Alcohol."

66. "Cancer and Food," *Lancet*, November 17, 1973; Berg, "Diet"; International Agency for Research on Cancer, *Annual Report 1975*.

67. Dr. Ernest L. Wynder quoted in *New York Times*, August 8, 1975; D. Mark Hegsted, "Summary of the Conference on Nutrition in the Causation of Cancer," *Cancer Research*, November 1975.

68. "Tackling Nutrition Problems in Africa," *WHO Chronicle*, Vol. 30, 1976, p. 29.

69. "Food and Nutrition Policies," *British Medical Journal*, August 21, 1976. See also Colin Blythe, "Eating Our Way Out of Debt and Disease," *New Scientist*, May 6, 1976; Colin Blythe, "Problems of Diet and Affluence," *Food Policy*, February 1976; and U.S. Senate, Select Committee on Nutrition and Human Needs, *Nutrition and Health II*, Committee Print, July 1976.

70. G. T. T. Molitor, "Anticipating Public Policy Issues: Nutrition, Diet, Health, and Food Quality," U. S. General Accounting Office, Washington, D. C., July 1976; National Board of Health and Welfare, *Diet and Exercise* (Stockholm: 1972); Royal Norwegian Ministry of Agriculture, "Report to the Storting No. 32 (1975-76) on Norwegian Nutrition and Food Policy," Oslo, November 7, 1975.

71. Hegsted, "Summary of the Conference."

63

ERIK ECKHOLM is a Senior Researcher with Worldwatch Institute. He is coauthor of *By Bread Alone* and author of *Losing Ground: Environmental Stress and World Food Prospects* (W.W. Norton, 1976). He is currently writing a book on environmental influences on health.

FRANK RECORD is a Researcher with Worldwatch Institute. He is a recent graduate of the Johns Hopkins University School of Advanced International Studies. Before joining Worldwatch, he worked as a Research Assistant for the World Bank.

THE WORLDWATCH PAPER SERIES

Worldwatch publications are available on a subscription basis for $25.00 a year. Subscribers receive all Worldwatch papers and books published during the calendar year for a single annual subscription. Single copies of Worldwatch Papers, including back copies, can be purchased for $2.00. Bulk copies are available at the following prices: 2-10 copies, $1.50 per copy; 11-50 copies, $1.25 per copy; and 51 or more copies, $1.00 per copy.

---

two dollars

Worldwatch Institute
1776 Massachusetts Avenue, N.W.
Washington, D.C. 20036 USA